Workbook for
Respiratory Disease
A Case Study Approach to Patient Care

Workbook for Respiratory Disease
A Case Study Approach to Patient Care

second edition

David W. Chang, EdD, RRT
Program Director/Professor
Department of Respiratory Therapy
Columbus College
Columbus, Georgia

Fred Corn, RRT
Respiratory Therapist
Phenix Regional Hospital
Phenix City, Alabama

 F. A. DAVIS COMPANY • Philadelphia

F. A. Davis Company
1915 Arch Street
Philadelphia, PA 19103

Printed in the United States of America

Last digit indicates print number: 10 9 8 7 6 5 4 3 2 1

Publisher, Health Professions: Jean-François Vilain
Senior Editor: Lynn Borders Caldwell
Developmental Editor: Marianne Fithian
Cover Designer: Louis J. Forgione

As new scientific information becomes available through basic and clinical research, recommended treatments and drug therapies undergo changes. The author and publisher have done everything possible to make this book accurate, up to date, and in accord with accepted standards at the time of publication. The author, editors, and publisher are not responsible for errors or omissions or for consequences from application of the book, and make no warranty, expressed or implied, in regard to the contents of the book. Any practice described in this book should be applied by the reader in accordance with professional standards of care used in regard to the unique circumstances that may apply in each situation. The reader is advised always to check product information (package inserts) for changes and new information regarding dose and contraindications before administering any drug. Caution is especially urged when using new or infrequently ordered drugs.

Preface

Research studies have clearly shown that learning is most likely to occur when there is active participation by students. Furthermore, self-learning can take place when the learning materials are organized in a logical manner and presented in small steps. When simple leading questions and immediate feedback are provided to the students, they are more likely to do their best in completing the task at hand. This workbook is written to make learning or reviewing respiratory diseases a more enjoyable experience for beginning students and seasoned RCPs.

This workbook uses many simple, but pertinent questions to help the students recall, interpret, and analyze the topics and concepts related to respiratory diseases. There are over 1400 questions in this workbook, ranging from simple multiple-choice questions to emphasize basic information to more challenging short-answer questions to reinforce important concepts. Students of respiratory disease should find this method of presentation very useful.

Users of this workbook should read the materials in each chapter of the textbook and then complete the questions in the workbook. This should be done soon after reading the chapter and case study but without frequently referring to the materials in the textbook. After completing all workbook questions for one chapter, the learner may verify the answers in the answer key and go on to another chapter.

Acknowledgments

We would like to thank our colleagues who provided insightful and practical guidance to our project. Their contributions have been invaluable in the development of this workbook. Our sincere gratitude goes out to the following individuals:

Thomas J. Butler, MS, RRT
Director of Clinical Education
Respiratory Care
Rockland Community College
Suffern, New York

Robert P. DeLorme, EdS, RRT
Division Chair
Health Sciences
Gwinnett Technical Institute
Lawrenceville, Georgia

Joanne Jacobs, MA, RRT
Department Chair
Cardiorespiratory Care Program
Community College of Rhode Island
Lincoln, Rhode Island

Paul J. Mathews, EdS, RRT
Associate Professor
Respiratory Care
University of Kansas Medical Center
Kansas City, Kansas

David J. Myers BS, RRT, CPFT
Former Program Director of Respiratory Care
Western School of Health and Business Careers
Pittsburgh, Pennsylvania

Mimi Yee Norwood, MA, MSW, RRT
Department Chair
Respiratory Therapy Program
Washtenaw Community College
Ann Arbor, Michigan

Drayton H. Odom, RRT
Director of Clinical Education
Respiratory Therapy
George C. Wallace Community College
Dothan, Alabama

Yvonne Jo Robbins, MEd, RRT
Program Director
Respiratory Therapy
West Chester University
West Chester, Pennsylvania

Peggy Spears, MS, RRT
Director of Clinical Education
Respiratory Therapy
Jefferson Community College
Louisville, Kentucky

Contents

CHAPTER 1

INTRODUCTION TO PATIENT ASSESSMENT

INTRODUCTION

1. Patient assessment is an important tool in patient care and it should be performed in which of the following setting(s): _____ .
   A. emergency room
   B. intensive care unit
   C. home-care setting
   D. A and B only
   E. A, B, and C

2. For a respiratory care practitioner (RCP), the purpose of patient assessment _is not_ (is, is not) to make a diagnosis, but to _assist_ (direct, assist) the physician in determining appropriate and effective therapy.

3. Describe the basic methods that should be included during pulmonary assessment.
   Chest x-ray, ABGs, chest ascultation, palpation, percussion, questions, examination (ascultation é viewing of film).

THE MEDICAL HISTORY AND THE INTERVIEW

4. List _five_ basic questions to ask the patient before performing physical assessment. _1. Where is problem? 2. Does it radiate?_
   1. How long has symptom occured?
   3. 2. How severe is the symptom?
   3. Does breathing affect symptom? what provokes; what makes better? what
   4. " occur " " " ?
   4. 5. When did problem start?
   5. 6. Have u had problem before?
5. Explain why the questions in answer 4 are important in the course of patient assessment.
   - differential diagnosis
   - further tests needed
   - initial therapy

1

6. List *seven* common symptoms that may be experienced by patients with cardiopulmonary disease.

1. *dyspnea*
2. *chest pain*
3. *fever*
5. *sputum*
6. *cough*
7. *wheezing*

7. Define dyspnea.
   Difficulty experienced w/ breathing *shortness of breath*

8. Shortness of breath that is worsened with exertion is called ___*exertional*___ dyspnea.

9. Patients with ___*poor*___ (good, poor) cardiopulmonary reserve will be dyspneic even at rest.

10. The type of shortness of breath that occurs only in the reclining (supine) position is called ___*orthopnea*___ .

11. Orthopnea is associated with ___*heart failure & lung disease*___ (heart failure only, lung disease only, heart failure and lung disease).

12. Platypnea refers to dyspnea in the ___*upright sitting*___ (prone, supine, upright) position.

13. List *four* types of cough receptors and for each receptor give at least one example that triggers the cough reflex.

1. *mechanical - dust particles*
2. *chemical - cigarette smoke*
3. *inflammation - of lung airways*
4. *thermal - cold*

14. Infection of the airways or pneumonia usually leads to a ___*productive*___ (dry, productive) cough whereas heart failure may be associated with a ___*dry*___ (dry, productive) cough.

15. A weak cough may indicate presence of all the following conditions **EXCEPT:** _____ .
    A. abdominal pain ✓
    B. neuromuscular disease ✓
    C. emphysema ✓
    D. bronchitis

16. to 19. Match the sputum terminologies with the characteristics. Use each answer *only once*.

Sputum Terminology	**Characteristic**
16. mucoid ___C___	A. foul smelling
17. fetid ___A___	B. large amount
18. purulent ___D___	C. clear and thick
19. copious ___B___	D. pus containing

20. Pleuritic chest pain is usually _____sharp_____ (dull, sharp) in nature and located laterally or posteriorly on the chest wall. This pain is often _____made worse_____ (relieved, made worse) by breathing deep.

21. Give *three* causes of pleuritic chest pain.

    1. pneumothorax
    2. pneumonia
    3. pulm. embolism

22. Nonpleuritic chest pain is more often located _____centrally_____ (laterally, centrally) in the chest because it is often associated with ischemic heart disease. It is usually _____unaffected_____ (affected, unaffected) by respiratory efforts.

23. Describe the sensations of nonpleuritic chest pain.

    Dull, radiates, pressure sensation to arm, back, jaw, shoulder

24. Define hemoptysis.

    The spitting up of blood

25. List at least *three* common causes of hemoptysis.

    1. pneumonia
    2. tuberculosis
    3. pulmonary embolism

26. _____Fever_____ (Wheezing, Chest pain, Hemoptysis, Fever) often occurs in response to an infection.

27. List at least *three* respiratory problems that lead to fever.

    1. Hyperventilation   bacterial bronchitis
    2. TB
    3. fungal infections

28. List *three* clinical conditions that may produce wheezing. bronchitis

    1. Obstruction of airway(s) - COPD
    2. asthma
    3. congestive heart failure

29. Wheezing is caused by _____rapid_____ (rapid, slow) airflow through one or more _____narrowed_____ (dilated, narrowed) airways.

30. Medical history of a patient is obtained to identify _____previously_____ (currently, previously) documented medical problems and findings.

PHYSICAL EXAMINATION

31. What are the *four* basic vital signs?

     1. RR

     2. BP

     3. HR

     4. Temperature

32. A rapid increase in heart rate above ___100___ beats per minute is known as tachycardia, whereas a decrease in the heart rate below ___60___ beats per minute is known as bradycardia.

33. A breathing rate higher than ___18___ per minute in the adult is known as tachypnea. The common causes of tachypnea are ___restrictive___ (obstructive, restrictive) disorders of the lung that have a reduction in lung ___volumes & capacities___ (flow rates, volumes and capacities).

34. Explain why reduction in lung volume causes tachypnea.

     In order to compensate for lost lung volumes RR's must be increased. To maintain MV c̄ reduced Vt

35. Name at least *three* pulmonary disorders that cause loss of lung volume.

     1. emphysema   pneumonia

     2. fibrosis   pulm oedema

     3. pulmonectomy   pulmon fibrosis

36. Bradypnea is a breathing rate less than ___10___ per minute and this condition may be seen with ___hypothermia___ (hyperthermia, hypothermia) or ___central___ (autonomic, central) nervous system disorders.

37. Hypothermia causes a(n) ___decrease___ (increase, decrease) in the amount of oxygen consumed and carbon dioxide produced by the body. This results in a(n) ___decrease___ (increased, reduced) need for breathing.

38. A complete lack of breathing is called ___apnea___ .

39. Normal arterial blood pressure of the systemic circulation is about ___120/80___ mm Hg in the adult patient. A measurement of less than ___90/60___ mm Hg is known as hypotension.

40. List *three* causes of severe hypotension.

     1. Decrease in heart rate

     2. Blood loss

     3. Dilation of vessels

41. Normal body temperature is about ___37___ °C or ___98.6___ °F.

42. Fever causes the metabolic rate of the patient to _increase_ (increase, decrease) slightly and this requires an _increase_ (increase, decrease) in the oxygen consumption and carbon dioxide production. As a result, this leads to a _higher_ (higher, lower) respiratory rate.

43. In hypothermia (temperature less than 32.5°C or 90°F), blood flow is shunted from the vital organs to systemic circulation. (True or False) _F_.

44. Explain the rationale for assessing a patient's sensorium.
By asking questions, O₂ (oxygenation status) to
brain is evaluated which reflects V and O.

45. During assessment of a patient's sensorium, a notation of "oriented ×3" means that the patient is alert to _name_, _location_, and _____.   t, place, person

46. Pulse oximetry loses its accuracy when the peripheral circulation is _inadequate_ (excessive, inadequate), and the measurements can be falsely _high_ (high, low) in the presence of carboxyhemoglobin (Hbco) or other dysfunctional hemoglobins.

47. Explain the differences in breathing patterns of patients with airway obstruction and those with lung restriction.
AO - long, deep breaths; prolonged e phase ;
sometimes i phase
LR - short, shallow breaths

48. Define abdominal paradox. What causes this observation?
As negative pressures are generated, the
abdomen is sucked upward and inward as
the diaphragm is incapable. (fatigued)

49. Asymmetrical chest expansion usually indicates _unilateral_ (unilateral, bilateral) chest diseases such as pneumonia or pneumothorax.

50. to 54. Match the chest wall deformities with the descriptions. Use each answer *only once*.

Chest Wall Deformity	*Description*
50. scoliosis ___B___	A. abnormal prominence of the sternum
51. kyphosis ___D___	B. lateral curvature of the spine
52. barrel chest ___E___	C. abnormal depression of the sternum
53. pectus excavatum ___C___	D. anterior-posterior curvature of the spine
54. pectus carinatum ___A___	E. increase in the anterior-posterior diameter of the chest

55. The tactile fremitus is increased when chest palpation is done over _consolidated_ (consolidated, air-filled) lung tissues. Explain why.
With a denser lung tissue, sounds better
heard (↑ tactile fremitus)

56. The tactile fremitus is _decreased_ (increased, decreased) when chest palpation is done over the lung tissues of patients with _pneumonia_ (emphysema, atelectasis, pneumonia).
emphysema

57. Describe the signs of subcutaneous emphysema.
A distinctive crackling sound is heard during chest palpation

58. Define diagnostic chest percussion.
Tapping on the chest wall in order to compare densities and resonating sounds.

59. Lung diseases that produce ___increased___ (increased, decreased) lung density such as pneumonia will result in ___decreased___ (increased, decreased) resonance on percussion.

60. Air trapped in the pleural space and emphysema cause ___increased___ (increased, decreased) resonance on percussion.

61. Breath sounds are assessed by doing ___chest auscultations___ .

62. The tracheal breath sound is heard directly over the ___trachea___ (mouth, trachea, main-stem bronchi) and has a ___loud___ and ___high pitched___ quality.

63. Bronchovesicular breath sounds are heard around the ___sternum___ on the ___anterior___ (anterior, lateral) chest wall and between the ___scapulas___ on the posterior chest wall.

64. Bronchovesicular breath sounds are ~~softer~~ ___louder___ (louder, softer) in intensity as compared with the tracheal breath sound and this sound is produced by ___turbulent___ (turbulent, laminar) flow in the larger airways.

65. Vesicular breath sounds are heard over the areas of the chest wall overlying ~~diseased~~ ___normal___ (normal, diseased) lung parenchyma and this sound is very ___soft___ (loud, soft) and primarily heard on ___inspiration___ (inspiration, expiration).

66. Harsh breath sounds heard on the chest wall over the diseased lung are called ___bronchial___ breath sounds.

67. Abnormal noises superimposed on the breath sounds are called ___adventitious___ lung sounds.

68. Wheezes resemble whistling sound and are most often heard during ___exhalation___ (inhalation, exhalation) because the airways become narrower during this phase.

69. ___Rhonchi___ (Rales, Rhonchi, Polyphonic wheezes) are sometimes called low-pitched wheezes.

70. Stridor is a wheezing-type breath sound most commonly heard during ___inspiration___ (inspiration, expiration) and this condition reflects ___partial___ (complete, partial) airway obstruction.

71. Discontinuous types of adventitious lung sounds are described as ___crackles___ or ___Rales___ .

72. Describe the *two* mechanisms that produce crackles.

At end inhalation, air pops open alveoli (atelectasis) _in smaller airways_
and fluid (pneumonia) build-up _excessive secretions w/_
breathing

73. Distension of the jugular vein may be indicative of __Rt__ (left, right) heart failure. Explain why.
Back-up of blood into PC and RV and
RA is indicated w/ distension of the
jugular vein.

74. Explain the differences between right ventricular heave and left anterior axillary heave. _w/ left ventricle failure_
Heave is in R and L ventricles on systolic
due to RV enlargement w/ abnormal pulsation - sternum

75. In a healthy heart, the first heart sound is produced by closure of the __mitral__ and __tricuspid__ valves during __systole__ (systole, diastole) while the second heart sound is produced by closure of the __pulmonary artery__ and __aorta__ valves during __diastole__ (systole, diastole).

76. In an abnormal or diseased heart, an additional sound known as __S³ gallop__ may be heard. This is caused by the sudden __filling__ (filling, emptying) of the ventricle with blood from the atrium during __diastole__ (systole, diastole).

77. Murmurs are adventitious heart sounds caused by __turbulent__ (smooth, turbulent) blood flow through a __narrow__ (wide, narrow) opening.

78. A bluish coloration of the skin from the presence of poorly __oxygenated__ (ventilated, oxygenated) blood is known as __cyanosis__.

79. An enlarged liver is called __hepatomegaly__. It is a sign of __R__ __right__ (left, right) ventricular failure.

80. Chronic left-sided heart failure or chronic lung disease may cause right ventricular failure. In turn, this may lead to hepatomegaly. (True or False) __T__.

81. Central cyanosis is a bluish coloration of the __oral__ mucosa and this condition indicates __severe__ (mild, moderate, severe) hypoxemia.

82. Explain why some patients breathe with pursed lips.
W/ obstructive disease, to produce a patent
airway for better V and therefore O.
— creates back pressure during exhalation;
maintains patency in distal airways.

LABORATORY DATA

83. Elevation of the white blood cell count to over __10,000__ per cubic millimeter is known as leukocytosis.

84. Decrease of the white blood cell count to less than __5000__ per cubic millimeter is called leukopenia.

85. Neutrophils are the most common __WBC__ (red blood cells, white blood cells, macrophages) and they are primarily responsible for fighting bacterial organisms.

86. The most common neutrophils are _____ segs _____ and _____ bands _____ .
_____ segs _____ are preferentially used for fighting infection. The immature ones
are called _____ bands _____ and when they are called into action, a relatively
_____ severe _____ (mild, severe) infection is present.

87. Surgery and hemorrhage are two common causes of _____ anemia _____ (leukopenia, leukocytosis, anemia, polycythemia).

88. Chronic hypoxia due to diseases and living at high altitude are two common causes of
_____ polycythemia _____ (leukopenia, leukocytosis, anemia, polycythemia).

89. Write the normal range for each of the following serum electrolytes: sodium (Na^+) potassium (K^+),
chloride (Cl^-), and total bicarbonate (HCO_3^-).

Na^+ 138 - 142 mEq/L
K^+ 3 - 5
Cl^- 101 - 105
HCO_3^- 23 - 27

90. The _____ culture Gram stain _____ (Gram stain, culture and sensitivity) method
helps to identify the general categories of microbes in a sputum sample and the
_____ Gram stain Culture sensitivity _____ (Gram stain, culture and sensitivity) method is used to
confirm the identity of microbes and the antibiotics that these microbes are sensitive to.

91. Acute injury to the myocardium causes the heart muscle cells to release _____ enzymes _____
(antibodies, fluid, sodium, enzymes) into the circulating blood. A(n) _____ elevated _____
(elevated, reduced) value of measurement is indicative of myocardial injury.

92. For adult patients, _____ severe _____ (mild, moderate, severe) hypoxemia is present when
the Pao_2 is below 40 mm Hg.

93. Elevation of the _____ $PaCO_2$ _____ ($Paco_2$, Pao_2) above 45 mm Hg is called hypercapnia. This is indicative
of _____ hypoventilation _____ (hyperventilation, hypoventilation, metabolic alkalo-
sis, metabolic acidosis).

94. Acidosis means a pH _____ below _____ (above, below) _____ 7.35 _____ . When this condition is caused by
_____ hypoventilation _____ (hyperventilation, hypoventilation), it is called respiratory acidosis.

95. Alkalosis means a pH _____ above _____ (above, below) _____ 7.45 _____ . When this condition is caused by
_____ hyperventilation _____ (hyperventilation, hypoventilation), it is called respiratory alkalosis.

96. Acidosis means a pH _____ (above, below) _____ . When this condition is caused by
_____ inadequate _____ (excessive, inadequate) bicarbonate, it is called metabolic acidosis.

97. Alkalosis means a pH _____ (above, below) _____ . When this condition is caused by
_____ excessive _____ (excessive, inadequate) bicarbonate, it is called metabolic alkalosis.

98. The amount of gas fully exhaled after a maximum inhalation is the _____ VC _____
(tidal volume, functional residual capacity, vital capacity, total lung capacity).

99. A forced expiratory volume in 1 second (FEV_1) of less than _____ 80% _____ predicted or
a forced expiratory flow during the middle half of the forced vital capacity ($FEF_{25-75\%}$) of less than
_____ 60% _____ predicted is indicative of obstructive lung disease.

100. Before and after bronchodilator pulmonary function tests (PFTs) are commonly done to evaluate the reversibility of _____*air flow obstruction*_____ (diffusion defect, restrictive lung disease, air flow obstruction).

101. List at least *three* clinical applications of chest radiographs.
     1. *Position of ETT*
     2. *" " nasogastric tube*
     3. *Disease of the lung (emphysema)*

102. Explain the method to evaluate the size of the heart using chest radiograph.
     Heart should be < one half of the entire chest cavity

103. Electrocardiogram (ECG) is a recording of the _____*electrical*_____ (mechanical, electrical) activity in the heart.

104. On a normal ECG tracing, the P wave signifies depolarization of the _____*atria*_____ (atria, ventricles).

105. The QRS complex on a normal ECG tracing occurs during _____*ventricular*_____ (atrial, ventricular) _____*depolarization*_____ (depolarization, repolarization).

106. The electrical activity during _____*atrial*_____ (atrial, ventricular) _____*repolarization*_____ (depolarization, repolarization) is not seen because it occurs at the same interval as _____*ventricular*_____ (atrial, ventricular) _____*depolarization*_____ (depolarization, repolarization).

107. On a normal ECG tracing, the PR interval should not be longer than _____*0.2*_____ second [5 small boxes on the ECG grid], a QRS complex should be no wider than _____*0.12*_____ second [3 small boxes on the ECG grid], and the ST segment should be relatively _____*flat*_____ (sine-wave shaped, flat).

108. A PR interval longer than 0.2 second is indicative of _____*1st degree heart block*_____ (first degree heart block, internal conduction defect, myocardial ischemia).

109. A widened QRS interval is a sign of _____*internal conduction defect*_____ (heart block, internal conduction defect, myocardial ischemia).

110. An elevated ST segment is a sign of myocardial _____*infarction / ischemia*_____

111. For patients with cardiac ischemia, describe the anticipated changes of the T waves, Q waves, and ST segments on an ECG tracing.
     T wave - elevated; inverted
     Q " - large (dead cells)
     ST segment - elevated

CHAPTER **2**

ETHICS IN RESPIRATORY CARE

INTRODUCTION

1. Changes in health care and medical technology have made the study of ethics in health care ___more___ (more, less) important and complicated.

CASE STUDY

2. The case study of Mrs. W. illustrated in this chapter deals with an ethical question concerning
   _____ .
   A. medical cost
   B. distribution of medical resources
   C. life support
   D. medical technology and advancement

3. Define ethics.
   moral convictions / virtues that govern decisions

4. The goal of ethics is to provide ___guidance___ (law and order, guidance) for living a virtuous life and for building a good society.

5. When ethics is applied to respiratory care, the goal is to state clearly how respiratory care practitioners (RCPs) should conduct their professional lives. (True or False) ___T___ .

6. List at least *three* factors that influence the development of a person's personal system of ethics and moral convictions.
   - _family / friends_
   - _society_
   - _education_

7. Taking direct action to end a person's life in a clinical setting is called _____ .
   A. homicide
   B. suicide
   C. active euthanasia
   D. passive euthanasia

8. Common morality refers to moral values of ___a society___ (an individual, a society) that are ___shared by others___ (unique to that person, shared by others).

9. Moral values are usually developed _____*gradually*_____ (rapidly, gradually) because the development is _____*frequently*_____ (frequently, seldomly) met with disagreements and controversies.

10. Professional ethics consists of the ethical convictions of a _____*specific*_____ (similar, specific) segment of society recognized as a profession.

11. Write the American Association for Respiratory Care (AARC) code of ethics on the following lines:

   _____

   _____

   _____

   _____

   _____

   _____

   _____

   _____

   _____

   _____

   _____

   _____

12. As stated in their respective codes of ethics, physicians, nurses, and RCPs are free to choose whom to serve. (True or False) _____*F*_____ .

13. When a member's incompetent, illegal, or unethical conduct is brought to light by a fellow member of the profession, it represents the profession's commitment to _____*self - regulation*_____ (perfection, truthfulness, self-regulation, prestige).

14. Which of the following statements shows that the code of ethics is used to establish society's trust in the profession? _____ .
   A. to guard against conflict of interest
   B. to provide best patient care with minimal resources
   C. to expose incompetent RCPs
   D. to treat all patients equal

15. Codes of ethics are sometimes insufficient. List *four* areas in which the codes of ethics may fall short of their intent.
   _____*refer to # 16 - #19*_____

   _____

   _____

   _____

16. Give an example to show why the codes of ethics may omit important norms and virtues.
   _____*Mrs. W wish to die is not*_____
   _____*being considered thy norms and virtues.*_____

17. Give an example to show why the codes of ethics are not extensive enough to anticipate and cover the complexity of all possible cases.

Mrs. W - use of sedatives, psych evaluation, and opposing decisions of family members.

18. Give an example to show why the codes of ethics cannot conform to the values of a changing society over time.

w/ drawing life support and use of sedatives to assist c euthenasia

19. Give an example to show why the codes of ethics may present conflicting rules.

Patient confidentiality and law cases may be an exception to the rule (a conflict of ethics)

ETHICAL PRINCIPLES

20. Define moral dilemma.

- when two or more moral conflicts come into conflict

21. A dilemma occurs when ___*two*___ (one, two) or more conflicting choice(s) are present.

22. Ethical principles are ___*broad*___ (broad, specific) statements of obligation that cover ___*large*___ (large, small) sectors of the moral obligation.

23. In ethics terminology, the right to govern self is called personal ___*autonomy*___ (decision, autonomy, choice, bias).

24. A patient's decision to terminate mechanical ventilation illustrates ___*personal autonomy*___.
    A. nonmaleficence
    B. moral principle
    C. euthanasia
    D. personal autonomy

25. To forbid or avoid deliberately injuring or harming a person is called ___*nonmaleficence*___.
    A. nonmaleficence
    B. beneficence
    C. paternalism
    D. principle of justice

26. The code of ethics that forbids RCPs to extend their practice beyond their competence is called ___*nonmaleficence*___

27. According to Beauchamp et al., it is more ethically problematic to ___*withdraw*___ (withhold, withdraw) artificial life support from a patient.

28. The code of ethics that is intended to increase and improve one's knowledge and skill illustrates the principle of _____ .
    A. nonmaleficence
    B. principle of justice
    C. beneficence
    D. paternalism

29. To override the wishes of a patient so as to provide what is best for the patient shows the principle of _____ .
    A. beneficence
    B. paternalism
    C. nonmaleficence
    D. principle of justice

30. Use at least one example to show that the need for paternalism in health care is a necessity.
    — when one is incompetent to making decisions
    — babies / small children

31. The principle of double effect usually involves decisions or actions that lead to _____ on the patient.
    A. two desirable effects
    B. one desirable effect and one harmful effect
    C. two harmful effects

32. The code of ethics that prescribes treatment be provided to patients unrestricted by considerations of social or economic status is based on the _____ .
    A. principle of justice
    B. principle of double effect
    C. principle of fidelity
    D. principle of beneficence

33. Discussing a patient's medical problem in public is a violation of the _____ .
    A. principle of fidelity
    B. principle of beneficence
    C. principle of double effect
    D. principle of justice

CHAPTER **3**

INTRODUCTION TO RESPIRATORY FAILURE

INTRODUCTION

1. Diffusion of oxygen through the alveolar capillary membrane into the blood of the pulmonary circulation is called ___external___ (internal, external) respiration.

2. ___Internal___ (Internal, External) respiration provides diffusion of oxygen into the systemic vascular tissue.

3. Besides oxygenating the blood, the lungs also serve to rid the body of ___CO_2___ a waste product of metabolism.

4. Failure of the cardiopulmonary system to provide and maintain adequate oxygenation for the blood is called ___respiratory___ (renal, ventilatory, respiratory) failure.

5. A patient has two sets of arterial blood gases (ABGs) within a 2-hour period. The results follow:

   ABG no. 1   pH 7.38
                        Pa_{CO_2} = 42 mm Hg
                        Pa_{O_2} = 74 mm Hg
                        F_{IO_2} = 35%
   ABG no. 2   pH 7.36
                        Pa_{CO_2} = 44 mm Hg
                        Pa_{O_2} = 53 mm Hg
                        F_{IO_2} = 55%

   This condition is known as ___ventilatory___ failure.

6. A patient has an admitting diagnosis of acute ventilatory failure. This is characterized by an increasing ___Pa_{CO_2}___ (Pa_{O_2}, Pa_{CO_2}) to a level higher than ___50___ mm Hg and a corresponding low pH (7.35 or lower).

ETIOLOGY

Oxygenation Failure

7. A patient's ABGs report shows a Pa_{O_2} value of 54 mm Hg. If the patient's normal Pa_{O_2} range is 80 to 100 mm Hg, the patient's oxygenation status is interpreted as ___hypoxemia___ (hypocapnia, acidosis, hypoxemia, hypokalemia).

8. Match the following Pa_{O_2} ranges with the proper interpretation of oxygenation status:

Oxygenation Status	*Pa_{O_2} Range (mm Hg)*
A. Mild hypoxemia	1. 80 to 100
B. Normal	2. 60 to 79
C. Moderate hypoxemia	3. 40 to 59
D. Severe hypoxemia	4. Less than 40

The preceding scale is for blood gases done on room air and for patients of less than ____60____ (40, 50, 60) years of age.

9. For patients over the age of ____60____ (50, 55, 60, 65), 1 mm Hg should be _____ (added, subtracted) from the predicted normal Pa_{O_2} for each year over 60.

[**NOTES**: Another way to do this is to add 1 mm Hg to the patient's actual Pa_{O_2} for each year of age over 60. For example, a 72-year-old patient with a Pa_{O_2} of 50 would have an "age-corrected" Pa_{O_2} of (72 – 60) + 50 equal to 62 mm Hg. The corrected Pa_{O_2} of 62 mm Hg is then used for interpreting a patient's oxygenation status. In this case, it is mild hypoxemia.]

10. A Pa_{O_2} of less than ____40____ mm Hg reflects severe hypoxemia at any age.

11. Match the following Pa_{O_2} values with the proper interpretation of oxygenation status (use age-corrected values for patients over 60 years of age):

Degree of Hypoxemia	*Age (yr)/Pa_{O_2} (mm Hg)*
A. normal	1. 45/57
B. mild	2. 57/77
C. moderate	3. 70/71
D. severe	4. 62/36

12. Hypoxia is defined as inadequate oxygenation ___at the tissues___ (in the lungs, in the blood, at the tissues) whereas hypoxemia is defined as inadequate oxygenation ___in the blood___ (in the lungs, in the blood, at the tissues).

13. A patient is suffering from moderate hypoxemia as documented by ABGs. You would expect the patient to compensate for this condition by (increasing, decreasing) ___increasing___ the cardiac output (heart rate and stroke volume).

14. The most common cause of hypoxemia is _____.
    A. $\dot{V}/\dot{Q}$ mismatch
    B. anatomic shunt
    C. hyperventilation
    D. low metabolic rate

15. Define low $\dot{V}/\dot{Q}$ (shunt). Explain how this occurs in the pulmonary system.

_____

_____

_____

_____

16. Define high $\dot{V}/\dot{Q}$ (dead space ventilation). Explain how this occurs in the pulmonary system.

_____

_____

_____

_____

17. Define intrapulmonary shunt. Explain how it causes hypoxemia.

_____

_____

18. A(n) ___physiologic___ (anatomic, physiologic) shunt often results from collapsed or unventilated alveoli.

19. An abnormal channel that allows venous blood to bypass the pulmonary circulation is an example of a(n) ___anatomic___ (anatomic, physiologic) shunt.

20. ___Hypoxemia___ can result from breathing a gas mixture of low partial pressure of oxygen. Two examples of situations when this condition can occur are ascending to high altitudes and combustion in an enclosed environment.

21. Hypoventilation ___decreases___ (increases, decreases) alveolar P_{O_2} (P_{AO_2}) and ___increases___ (increases, decreases) alveolar P_{CO_2} (P_{ACO_2}).

22. Hypoventilation on room air can cause hypoxemia. This type of hypoxemia may be corrected by increasing the level of ventilation or ___FiO_2___ .

Ventilatory Failure

23. Contraction of the diaphragm and inhalation occur when the intrathoracic pressure is ___decreased___ (increased, decreased).

24. The work of breathing is normal when the chest cage is intact, airways are ___patent___ (patent, constricted), and lungs are ___compliant___ (compliant, noncompliant).

25. Normal exhalation requires patent airways and proper level of ___elastic recoil___ (airflow resistance, elastic recoil) in the lungs.

26. Match the following patient conditions with the type of systemic dysfunctions leading to ventilatory failure (you may use any answer more than once):

Type of Dysfunction

A. central nervous system 2, 6
B. neuromuscular
C. musculoskeletal 5
D. pulmonary 3, 8

Patient Condition

1. myasthenia gravis
2. drug overdose
3. emphysema
4. Guillain-Barré
5. chest trauma
6. head injury
7. sleep apnea (central or obstructive)
8. asthma

27. A chronic obstructive pulmonary disease (COPD) patient has chronic air trapping and lung hyperinflation. You would expect the patient's diaphragm to assume an abnormally __low__ (high, low) position that can result in the impairment of ventilation and gas exchange.

28. Due to air trapping, a common problem with COPD patients is lung __hyperinflation__ (collapse, hyperinflation, hyperventilation).

PATHOPHYSIOLOGY

Oxygenation Failure

29. The _____ (type, severity) of hypoxemia and the patient's preexisting condition will determine the response to hypoxemia.

30. The most common response to hypoxemia is a(n) _____ (increased, decreased) rate of breathing. This condition usually causes a(n) _____ (increased, decreased) minute volume, _____ (increased, decreased) P_{ACO_2}, and an _____ (increased, decreased) P_{AO_2}.

31. Define anatomic dead space.

    _____

    _____

32. Alveolar hypoxia causes the pulmonary capillaries to __constrict__ (dilate, constrict) in the affected regions. This is known as __vasoconstriction__ (vasodilation, vasoconstriction).

33. Pulmonary vasoconstriction leads to a(n) __increased__ (increased, decreased) vascular resistance and work load of the __R__ (right, left) heart.

34. Pumping blood against the constricted pulmonary capillaries will increase the __R__ (left, right) heart pressures.

35. Cor pulmonale means __R__ (left, right) heart or ventricular failure caused by chronic lung disease and pulmonary hypertension.

36. Two compensatory mechanisms for hypoxemia are __increased__ (increased, decreased) heart rate and __increased__ (increased, decreased) myocardial contraction.

37. The effects on the brain caused by severe hypoxemia or inadequate cardiac output are a diminished _____ and cognitive functions. If the brain continues to be hypoxic, the patient will lose consciousness and lapse into a __coma__.

Ventilatory Failure

38. In patients with acute ventilatory failure, you would expect to see a(n) __decreased__ (normal, increased, decreased) arterial blood pH and __increased__ (normal, increased, decreased) P_{ACO_2}.

39. Cerebral and peripheral blood vessels react to hypercapnia by _____ (vasodilation, vasoconstriction), thus providing more perfusion to the vital organs such as the brain.

CLINICAL FEATURES

Oxygenation Failure

40. One of the common clinical features of severe hypoxemia is the use of _____*accessory*_____ muscles. This indicates an increased work of _____*breathing*_____ .

41. A bluish appearance of the tongue and mucous membranes is called central _____*hypoxia*_____ . This condition is caused by the desaturation of hemoglobin and it may be difficult to detect if _____*anemia*_____ (polycythemia, hyperoxia, anemia, hypoxia) is present.

42. The vital signs of a patient with severe hypoxemia are typically abnormal and may demonstrate all the following **EXCEPT**: _____ .
    A. tachycardia
    B. respiratory arrest
    C. tachypnea

43. Confusion and agitation may be seen in patients with severe hypoxemia. This is due to the effects of
    _____ .
    A. cerebral hypoxia
    B. hepatomegaly
    C. cor pulmonale
    D. hyperventilation

44. Chronic hypoxemia causes a persistent _____*increase*_____ (increase, decrease) of pulmonary vascular resistance. This change in pulmonary vascular resistance can lead to _____*R*_____ (left, right) heart failure or cor pulmonale. Symptoms of this condition may include all the following **EXCEPT**:
    _____ .
    A. digital clubbing
    B. pedal edema
    C. hepatomegaly
    D. bronchospasm
    E. loud pulmonic valve closing

45. In chronic hypoxemia, ABGs and blood component parameters will change according to the degree of hypoxemia. Match the parameters with the type of change, if any (you may use any answer more than once):

Blood Gas Parameters	Type of Changes in Chronic Hypoxemia
A. Pa_{O_2} ↓	1. Increase
B. Sa_{O_2} ↓	2. Decrease
C. Hematocrit	3. No change
D. Hemoglobin 3	

46. Polycythemia results when chronic hypoxemia stimulates bone marrow to produce excess _____*red*_____ (red, white) blood cells.

47. Polycythemia can compensate for hypoxemia and hypoxia because the vast majority of oxygen carried by the blood is attached to the _____*Hb*_____ . Therefore, the arterial oxygen content (Ca_{O_2}) may be normal or near normal in the presence of long-standing low Pa_{O_2}.

48. With oxygenation failure the chest radiograph may show abnormalities such as infiltrates. This would be consistent with all of the following conditions **EXCEPT**: _____.
    A. pulmonary edema
    B. adult respiratory distress syndrome
    C. atelectasis
    D. pneumonia
    E. asthma

Ventilatory Failure

49. All the following clinical findings may suggest ventilatory failure with the **EXCEPTION** of: _____
    _____.
    A. headache
    B. diminished alertness
    C. hyperventilation
    D. warm flushed skin, and bounding peripheral pulses

50. When ventilatory failure is caused by sedative overdose _hypothermia_
    (hypothermia, hyperthermia) and _loss of consciousness_ (excitability, loss of
    consciousness) are two common findings.

51. _Fixed & dilated_ (Fixed and dilated, Reactive and constricted) pupils are
    the sign of drug overdose from sedatives or tricyclic antidepressants.

52. Aspiration is likely in sedative and alcohol abuse because of a diminished _gag_
    (gag, swallow) reflex. When aspiration occurs, _crackles_ (crackles, stridor, wheez-
    ing) may be heard in the lower lobes, particularly the _R_ (left, right) lower lobe.

53. Tachypnea, respiratory alternans, or abdominal paradox are signs of fatigue of the _____
    diaphragm.

54. An elevated _PaCO_2_ (pH, P_{aCO_2}, P_{aO_2}) in conjunction with a low _pH_ (pH, P_{aCO_2}) are
    signs of ventilatory failure. Immediate respiratory intervention is indicated when the pH is lower than 7.20.

TREATMENT

Oxygenation Failure

55. The initial treatment for hypoxemia should be _PEEP_ (mechan-
    ical ventilation, oxygenation, PEEP).

56. A patient has a diagnosis of pneumonia. The ABGs show moderate hypoxemia due to $\dot{V}/\dot{Q}$ mismatch. This
    type of hypoxemia can readily be corrected by _____
    CPAP (oxygen therapy, intermittent positive pressure breathing [IPPB],
    CPAP, PEEP).

57. The following blood gas results are obtained from a 45-year-old patient diagnosed with acute bronchitis:
    pH = 7.36, P_{CO_2} = 45 mm Hg, P_{O_2} = 56 mm Hg, and F_{IO_2} = 21 percent. The interpretation is _moderate_
    (mild, moderate, severe) hypoxemia with mild _hypoventilation_ (hyperventilation, hypoven-
    tilation). This type of hypoxemia can readily be corrected by _____
    _____ (CPAP, PEEP, pressure support ventilation, oxygen therapy).

58. A physician asks you to select the proper oxygen therapy device for a patient who requires precise oxygen concentrations. You would recommend a _____Venturi mask_____ (nasal cannula, simple mask, Venturi mask).

59. The F_{IO_2} of a nasal cannula and simple mask may vary depending on the patient's _____RR_____ _____breathing pattern_____ and _____breathing pattern_____.

60. Hypoxemia caused by anatomic or physiologic shunts _____does not_____ (does, does not) readily respond to an increased F_{IO_2}. This is because _____ventilation is not occurring; perfusion cannot occur_____

61. Treatment of _____anatomic_____ (anatomic, physiologic) shunts requires closure of the defect.

62. Treatment of _____physiologic_____ (anatomic, physiologic) shunts requires re-opening of the alveoli or reestablishing the functional residual capacity (FRC).

63. Collapsed alveoli or reduced FRC usually responds to treatment by _____ _____ .

64. The ABGs of a patient show: Pa_{CO_2} = 58 mm Hg, Pa_{O_2} = 43 mm Hg, F_{IO_2} = 60%.
    A. To improve the blood gases, should the next step be increasing the Fio2 only?
    B. If no is the anwer to question A, what type of treatment is indicated?

    _____

65. What does CPAP stand for?

    _____

66. CPAP is an appropriate mode of treatment for patients who are _____able_____ (able, unable) to maintain adequate ventilation.

67. Give *three* conditions under which mask CPAP should be changed to intubation and mechanical ventilation.

    _____

    _____

    _____

68. What does PEEP stand for?

    _____

69. PEEP or CPAP provides oxygenation at a _____↓_____ (higher, lower) F_{IO_2}, thus reducing the risk of _____O_2 toxicity_____ .

70. What does IMV stand for? _____Intermittent Mandatory Ventilation_____ .

71. During mechanical ventilation an _____IMV_____ (assist control, IMV) mode allows the patient to take spontaneous breaths, while in an _____assist control_____ (assist control, IMV) mode the patient's inspiratory effort results in a mechanical breath.

72. With traditional methods of mechanical ventilation the _____ (inspiratory, expiratory) time is usually shorter than the _____ (inspiratory, expiratory) time.

73. As you are monitoring a patient on the mechanical ventilator, you notice that the 67-year-old COPD patient has air trapping. You may minimize this problem by using a longer _____ _____ (inspiratory, expiratory) time on the ventilator. This can be done by _____ (increasing, decreasing) the inspiratory flow rate.

74. Patients with poor gas exchange due to very low *lung compliance* _____ (lung compliance, airway resistance) may benefit from an inverse inspiratory time to expiratory time (I:E) ratio.

75. Inverse-ratio ventilation (IRV) can be used successfully in adult patients with _____ _____ (hyperventilation, hypotension, refractory hypoxemia).

Ventilatory Failure

76. An elevation of arterial ___PCO_2___ (pH, Po_2, Pco_2) is an indication that the patient cannot maintain adequate alveolar ventilation.

77. The clinical guidelines for initiation of mechanical ventilation for adult patients include
    A. spontaneous respiratory rate greater than _____ (25, 35) breaths per minute
    B. vital capacity less than _____ (15, 25, 30, 35) cc/kg
    C. spontaneous minute ventilation greater than _____ (5, 8, 10) liters/minute for acceptable blood gases
    D. maximum inspiratory pressure less than _____ (–5, –10, –20) cm H_2O
    E. $Paco_2$ greater than ___50___ (30, 40, 50) mm Hg
    F. Pao_2 less than ___60___ (60, 70, 80) mm Hg

78. A physician asks you to set the tidal volume (V_T) of a mechanical ventilator for an adult patient. You would suggest setting the V_T in the range of ___10___ to ___15___ cc/kg of ideal body weight. If the patient weighs 60 kg (132 lb), the V_T should be in the range of ___500___ to ___600___ mL.

79. As you verify the physician's order for the settings of a mechanical ventilator, you notice that the order reads "V_T 20 cc/kg." You would explain to the physician that V_T for mechanical ventilation greater than 10 to 15 cc/kg may cause excessive inspiratory pressure, and _____ may result.
    A. atelectasis
    B. pneumothorax
    C. pneumomediastinum
    D. A and B only
    E. B and C only

80. V_Ts less than 10 to 15 cc/kg may cause ___atelectasis___ (atelectasis, pneumothorax, pneumediastinum, air trapping).

81. In mechanical ventilation, the ventilator rate and V_T are usually adjusted to maintain the $Paco_2$ between ___35___ and ___45___ mm Hg. One exception is for the patient with cerebral edema, where a lower $Paco_2$ is needed to lower the ___intracranial___ pressure.

82. The goal of mechanical ventilation for patients with chronic CO_2 retention (elevated $Paco_2$ and HCO_3-) is to _____ .
    I. return the pH to patient's normal
    II. increase the minute ventilation
    III. return the $Paco_2$ to patient's normal baseline values
    IV. reduce the patient's maximum inspiratory pressure

    A. I and III only
    B. I and IV only
    C. I, II, and III only
    D. II, III, and IV only

83. In patients with chronic hypoventilation and CO_2 retention it is not desirable to ventilate to normal $Paco_2$ values (35 to 45 mm Hg) because ____alkalosis____ (acidosis, alkalosis) can result and make weaning difficult.

84. A patient in the emergency department has a diagnosis of drug overdose. The nonpulmonary management protocols for this patient would include

    _____

    _____

    _____

85. Once the cause of ventilatory failure has been corrected and the patient stabilized, weaning from mechanical ventilation may be evaluated using the following criteria:
    A. vital capacity greater than _____ (5 to 10, 7 to 12, 10 to 15) ml/kg
    B. resting minute volume less than _____ (10, 15, 20, 25) liters/minute to maintain satisfactory blood gases
    C. maximum inspiratory pressure greater than _____ (−5, −10, −20) cm H_2O
    D. adequate oxygenation on Fio_2 less than _____ (0.50, 0.60, 0.70, 0.80)
    E. spontaneous respiratory rate less than _____ (35, 40, 45) breaths per minute to maintain satisfactory blood gases
    F. minimum spontaneous V_T of _____ (225, 325) cc

86. ____PS____ (IMV, Pressure support, T-piece weaning) helps to overcome the resistance of the artificial airway and ventilator circuit by maintaining an appropriate level of positive pressure during _____ (expiration, inspiration).

87. A physician wants to use the weaning process in which the number of mechanical breaths is decreased gradually until mechanical support is no longer needed. You would initiate the __IMV__ _____ (IMV, pressure support, T-piece) technique.

88. Alternating mechanical ventilation and spontaneous breathing with increasing periods of spontaneous breathing best describes ____T-piece____ (IMV, pressure support, T-piece) weaning.

89. One disadvantage of the ventilator demand valve is that it increases the work of breathing during delivery of ____spontaneous____ (spontaneous, mechanical) breaths in the IMV mode.

CHAPTER **4**

ASTHMA

INTRODUCTION

1. Asthma is a(n) _obstructive_ (obstructive, restrictive) pulmonary disease characterized by diffuse _bronchospasms_ (bronchospasms, lung infiltrates).

2. A key feature of asthma is that the airway obstruction is _reversible_ (reversible, irreversible).

3. When a patient's asthma attack does not respond to conventional treatment the condition is called _status asthmaticus_ .

4. Match the type of asthma with the major classification (intrinsic or extrinsic) as follows:

Classification	Type of Asthma
A. intrinsic	1. occurs commonly in childhood
B. extrinsic	2. starts in adult life
	3. caused by irritants
	4. not caused by irritants

5. Bronchospasms brought on by an irritant in the work place is called _occupational_ (occupational, bronchial, congenital) asthma.

6. Stable asthma is when the patient experiences no deterioration in symptoms or medications for about _1 month_ (1 week, 1 month, 3 months, 1 year).

ETIOLOGY

7. Asthma attacks may be brought on by different causes. Match the specific cause of asthma with the corresponding type of trigger. You may use any answer *more than once*.

Type of Trigger	Cause of Asthma
A. drugs 2,	1. sulfur dioxide
B. air pollution 3, 1, 8	2. aspirin
C. exercise induced 7	3. cigarette smoke
D. allergens 4, 6, 5,	4. certain food
	5. house dust mites
	6. food additives
	7. physical activities
	8. oxidants

PATHOPHYSIOLOGY

8. Airway obstruction in asthma may be caused by _____ .
   I. bronchospasms ✓
   II. mucosal edema ✓
   III. excessive secretions ✓
   IV. bilateral lung infiltrates

   A. I and II only
   (B.) I, II, and III only
   C. II and III only
   D. II, III, and IV only

9. Patients with asthma frequently have _____thick_____ (thick, thin) secretions in the lungs causing _____obstruction_____ of the distal airways.

10. Airway obstruction in asthma hinders exhalation and leads to _____ .
    _____ .
    I. air trapping ✓
    II. progressive lung inflation
    III. hyperinflation ✓
    IV. decreased airway resistance

    A. I and II only
    (B.) I, II, and III only
    C. II and III only
    D. III and IV only

11. Air trapping _____increases_____ (increases, decreases) the residual volume. As a result, the vital capacity _____decreases_____ (increases, decreases).

12. _____High_____ (High, Low) airway resistance and hyperinflation of the lungs cause the work of breathing to be _____increased_____ (increased, decreased).

CLINICAL FEATURES

Medical History

13. Patients having an asthma attack usually complain of chest tightness, difficulty breathing, and wheezing or cough (or both). (True or False) _____T_____ .

14. The severity of an asthma attack can be determined by the degree of dyspnea. (True or False) _____F_____ .

15. Dyspnea and wheezing are diagnostic of asthma. (True or False) _____F_____ .

16. Diagnosis of asthma can best come from the patient's age, medical history, physical findings, and radiographic and laboratory results. (True or False) _____T_____ .

Physical Examination

17. Physical examination of an asthma patient provides objective information to confirm the _____diagnosis_____ (diagnosis, prognosis) of asthma and identify the severity of airway obstruction.

18. The physical findings of asthma include (1) _rapid_ (rapid, slow) respiratory rate, (2) _active_ (active, inactive) use of accessory muscles for breathing, (3) prolonged _inhalation_ (inhalation, exhalation), (4) _increased_ (increased, decreased) anteroposterior diameter of the chest, (5) _presence_ (presence, absence) of wheezing, and (6) _retraction_ (relaxation, retraction) of the intercostal muscles.

19. In asthma, the expiratory phase is usually _prolonged_ (prolonged, shortened) due to airway obstruction.

20. An increased anteroposterior diameter (AP) of the chest is found when _____ _____ are present.
    I. dyspnea
    II. pulmonary hyperinflation ✓
    III. tachypnea
    IV. air trapping ✓

    A. I and III only
    B. I and V only
    C. II and III only
    D. II and IV only ⃝

21. _Wheezing_ (Wheezing, Stridor, Crackles, Rales) is an abnormal breath sound produced during movement of rapid airflow through the narrowed airways. This "musical" breath sound can sometimes be heard without a stethoscope.

22. Define retractions. What does this sign indicate?
    - depressed of skin around ribs on i phase
    - WOB is high w/ airway obstruction with
    low lung compliance (or chest wall)

23. Chest retractions are caused by a significant _negative_ (positive, negative) intrapleural pressure.

24. The decrease in intrapleural pressure is responsible for the drop in pulse pressure during _inspiration_ (inspiration, expiration). This is called a _paradoxical_ pulse.

Laboratory Evaluation

25. In the absence of complications, the chest radiograph of asthma typically shows _hyper-inflation_ (atelectasis, hyperinflation) of the lungs.

26. In the evaluation of asthma, bedside spirometry is useful for determining the _____ _____.
    I. severity of obstructions ✓
    II. residual volume
    III. response to therapy
    IV. level of hypoxemia ✓

    A. I and III only ⃝
    B. I and IV only
    C. II and III only
    D. II and IV only

27. FEV_1 stands for ___forced expiratory volume___ .

28. A peak flow of less than ___100___ (1, 10, 100) liters/minute or FEV_1 of less than ___1___ (1, 10, 100) liter(s) suggests severe airway obstruction.

29. Bronchial provocation, a pulmonary function test involving methacholine, is used to identify the degree of ___reactivity___ .

30. Methacholine ___increases___ (increases, decreases) the parasympathetic tone of smooth muscle. When the parasympathetic system is ___stimulated___ (stimulated, inhibited), ___bronchospasm___ (bronchospasm, bronchodilation) results.

31. At an effective dose of methacholine, patients with asthma will show a 20 percent or more ___decrease___ (increase, decrease) in FEV_1.

32. At the onset of an asthma attack arterial blood gases (ABGs) typically show a(n) ___decreased___ (increased, decreased, normal) $Paco_2$.

33. If the airway obstruction in asthma is severe or the patient is becoming fatigued, the $Paco_2$ will be normal or ___increased___ (increased, decreased).

TREATMENT

34. The initial treatment protocol for asthma should include _____ .
    I. oxygenation ✓
    II. bronchodilators ✓
    III. testing for airway reactivity
    IV. reduction of airway inflammation ✓

    A. I, II, and III
    B. I, II, and IV
    C. I, III, and IV
    D. II, III, and IV

35. β_2-Adrenergics, xanthines, and parasympatholytics are some medications that promote ___bronchodilation___ . Steroids are used to decrease airway ___inflammation___ .

36. In comparison between inhaled and oral bronchodilators, the ___inhaled___ route has the following advantages: rapid onset, lower dosage, fewer side effects, and better protection of the airways against provoking agents.

37. MDI stands for ___Metered Dose Inhaler___ .

38. MDI is common among patients with asthma or airway obstruction because it is ___convenient___ (convenient, inexpensive) to use.

39. SVN stands for ___Small Volume Nebulizer___ .

40. SVN treatments are usually given every ___4___ to ___6___ hours.

41. Candidates for oral or intravenous ___theophylline___ are patients who fail to respond to aerosolized β-agonist or who have severe asthma.

42. The anti-inflammatory effects of corticosteroids for asthma may not be apparent for several ___hours___ (minutes, hours, days).

43. A patient should not be given sedatives during an asthma attack because sedatives can induce ___ventilatory___ failure.

44. Mucomyst, cromolyn sodium, and dense aerosols (e.g., ultrasonic nebulizer) should not be given to the patient during an asthma attack because they may increase the incidence of ___broncho-spasm___ (bronchospasm, cardiac arrhythmia).

45. ___Hydration___ (Dehydration, Hydration) of the airways and lungs helps the patient to expectorate the pulmonary secretions.

46. The patient should be admitted to the hospital if the asthma causes the following symptoms:
    A. use of accessory muscles ___at rest___ (during exercise, at rest)
    B. paradoxic pulse ___present___ (present, absent)
    C. inspiratory and expiratory wheezing ___present___ (present, absent)
    D. peak flow less than ___100___ (1, 10, 100) liters/minute
    E. ___hyperinflation___ (atelectasis, hyperinflation) on chest radiograph

    The patient is not responding to initial therapy for asthma when the following signs are observed:
    F. continued use of ___accessory___ muscles
    G. Pao$_2$ responds minimally to ___oxygen___ therapy

47. The patient should be intubated and mechanically ventilated if the patient fatigues and these criteria are met (write in the following changes):
    A. ___↑___ Paco$_2$
    B. ___↓___ sensorium
    C. ___presence___ of abdominal paradox
    D. ___↓___ peak flow

    Respiratory failure is present when the following signs are observed:
    E. hypoxemia despite high ___oxygenation or FiO$_2$___
    F. respiratory acidemia (pH ___is less than 7.25___)
    G. central cyanosis is ___present___

    Cardiopulmonary arrest is evident when the following signs are observed:
    H. pulse and respiratory effort ___absent___
    I. pallor ___present___
    J. patient becomes ___unconscious___

48. Preventing or reducing the incidence of asthma attacks is done by ___decreasing___ airway responsiveness.

49. Patient education on asthma should include ___avoidance___ (avoidance, inclusion) of provoking agents, use of ___medications___ (medications, accessory muscles), and management of the side effects of medications.

50. The ___peak flow meter___ (peak flow meter, incentive spirometer) can be used by the patient to monitor the degree of airway obstruction. This can help the patient to adjust the medication dose and to seek medical attention.

51. Cromolyn sodium stabilizes the _____mast_____ (mast, bronchial) cells that release mediators such as _____histamine_____ (heparin, histamine) that can cause _____broncho spasm_____ (bronchospasm, bronchodilation).

CHAPTER **5**

CHRONIC BRONCHITIS

INTRODUCTION

1. Chronic bronchitis is a pulmonary disease in which the patient has a long-standing _____ _____ (productive, nonproductive) cough due to inflamed airways, particularly the bronchi.

2. The criteria for chronic bronchitis are the presence of a productive cough at least _____ (3, 4, 6) consecutive months of the year for _____ (2, 3, 4) successive years.

3. COPD stands for _____ .

4. The majority of COPD patients have a combination of
   I. asthma
   II. chronic bronchitis
   III. emphysema
   IV. cystic fibrosis (CF)

   A. I and II
   B. I and III
   C. II and III
   D. III and IV

5. Which disease is **NOT** included under the heading of COPD?
   A. asthma
   B. chronic bronchitis
   C. emphysema
   D. pneumonia

ETIOLOGY

6. The major contributing factor in the development of chronic bronchitis is _____ _____ .

7. Name *three* other contributing factors of chronic bronchitis.

   _____

   _____

   _____

PATHOLOGY AND PATHOPHYSIOLOGY

8. In chronic bronchitis an increase in mucus production is usually seen. This is because the size of bronchial mucous glands is _____ (larger, smaller) than normal and the number of goblet cells is _____ (higher, lower) than normal.

9. Continued exposure to cigarette smoke causes the lungs to retain secretions because of excessive mucus production and diminished function of the _____ (cilia, goblet cells, macrophages).

10. Mucus plugging is a result of excessive _____ production and _____ loss.

11. Inflammation and excessive secretions in the airways lead to reduced _____ (airflow, elasticity, airway resistance) in chronic bronchitis.

12. Ventilation-perfusion ($\dot{V}/\dot{Q}$) mismatch usually causes _____ (hypoxemia, pulmonary vasodilation, respiratory failure).

13. Hypoxemia leads to hypoxic _____ (vasoconstriction, vasodilation) of the pulmonary vasculature.

14. Acidosis causes _____ (dilation, constriction) of the pulmonary blood vessels.

15. Hypoxemia and acidosis _____ (increase, decrease) the blood pressure in the pulmonary circulation resulting in a condition known as pulmonary _____ (hypertension, hypotension).

16. Pulmonary hypertension _____ (increases, decreases) the work of the _____ (left, right) heart.

17. If pulmonary hypertension is persistent and left uncorrected _____ (right, left) heart failure will occur eventually. This condition is known as _____ .

CLINICAL FEATURES

Medical History

18. Chronic bronchitis patients often report _____ and _____ production.

19. In uncomplicated chronic bronchitis the mucus can be _____ in color.
A. brown
B. bloody
C. white or mucoid
D. yellow-green

20. After performing aerosol therapy and chest physiotherapy to a patient with chronic bronchitis and pneumonia, the patient coughs up a moderate amount of sputum. On examination of the sputum, you would expect it to be thick, purulent, and _____ (yellow-green, white, mucoid, brown) in color.

21. Coughing up blood is called _____ .

Physical Examination

22. With severe chronic bronchitis or during acute exacerbations of chronic bronchitis, physical examination may reveal several distinct findings. Match the following clinical signs with the significance:

Clinical Signs	*Suggested Significance*
A. coarse crackles	1. infection present
B. expiratory wheezes	2. pulmonary hypertension
C. jugular vein distension	3. excessive airway secretions
D. loud pulmonic valve closure	4. airway obstruction
E. fever	5. cor pulmonale

23. In chronic bronchitis, the accessory muscles for breathing _____ (are, are not) used and the respiratory cycle may show a prolonged _____ (inspiratory, expiratory) phase. These two signs _____ (are, are not) consistent with the presence of airway obstruction.

24. Cor pulmonale may lead to all the following conditions with the **EXCEPTION** of: _____
_____ .

    A. jugular vein distension
    B. pedal edema
    C. pulmonary edema
    D. hepatomegaly

25. The immediate clinical signs of severe hypoxemia and hypercapnia include _____
_____ .

    I. cyanosis of the tongue and mucous membranes
    II. jugular vein distension
    III. increased mucus production
    IV. disorientation and confusion

    A. I and II
    B. I, II, and III
    C. I and IV
    D. II, III, and IV

Laboratory Evaluation

26. Chronic hypoxemia may increase the production of _____ (red, white) blood cells. This is done to increase the carrying capacity of _____ (oxygen, carbon dioxide) in blood.

27. The _____ (red blood cell, white blood cell, platelet) count is usually elevated if infection is present.

28. In severe chronic bronchitis, arterial blood gases (ABGs) usually show _____ (hypoxemia, hypocapnia) along with respiratory _____ (acidosis, alkalosis).

29. An enlarged right heart border on the chest radiograph indicates the presence of _____
_____ .

30. In severe chronic bronchitis the expiratory flow rates and vital capacity are typically _____ _____ (increased, decreased) whereas the residual volume is _____ (increased, decreased).

31. Patients with chronic bronchitis (i.e., in the absence of any component of emphysema) usually have _____ (diminished, normal, elevated) total lung capacity and _____ (diminished, normal, elevated) gas diffusion capacity.

32. Ms. Oakley, a 75-year-old patient with an admitting diagnosis of chronic bronchitis and cor pulmonale, is being treated in the coronary care unit for chest pain. On her daily electrocardiograph, you would expect to see _____ .
    A. left bundle branch block
    B. right axis deviation
    C. ventricular fibrillation
    D. atrial tachycardia

TREATMENT

33. The general goals in the management of chronic bronchitis are to _____ _____ .
    I. decrease the lung compliance
    II. slow the progression of disease
    III. increase the residual volume
    IV. treat all acute medical problems

    A. I and II
    B. I and IV
    C. II and III
    D. II and IV

34. Nicotine polacrilex (gum) and transdermal nicotine patches can be used to manage the symptoms of _____ withdrawal.

35. When infection and acute bronchospasm are present, all the following medications may be helpful with the **EXCEPTION** of: _____ .
    A. cromolyn sodium
    B. antibiotics
    C. sympathomimetic bronchodilators
    D. corticosteroid
    E. theophylline

36. Mr. Kingsley, a 45-year-old patient with a history of chronic bronchitis, is being treated for pneumonia. The physician asks you to perform respiratory care procedures for removal of excessive secretions. In addition to bronchodilator and mucolytic agents, you would recommend _____ _____ .
    A. postural drainage
    B. endotracheal intubation
    C. nasotracheal suction
    D. bronchoscopy

37. A physician asks you if Mr. Kingsley needs any oxygen. You would answer that supplemental oxygen is indicated when the Pa_{O_2} done on room air approaches _____ (35, 45, 55) mm Hg.

38. The oxygen flow rate to be administered to Mr. Kinsley should be titrated by using the _____ (arterial, venous, mixed venous) _____ (pH, P_{CO_2}, P_{O_2}) value.

CHAPTER **6**

EMPHYSEMA

INTRODUCTION

1. Emphysema is a(n) _____ (obstructive, restrictive) lung disease characterized by _____ (dilation, constriction) and destruction of the lung structures from the terminal _____ (bronchi, bronchioles) to the alveoli.

2. Panlobular emphysema is a form of emphysema that causes enlargement of all airspaces distal to the terminal bronchioles, _____ (including, excluding) the respiratory bronchioles, alveolar ducts, and alveoli. Panlobular emphysema is commonly caused by a hereditary _____ _____ (deficiency, excess) of α_1-protease inhibitor (α_1PI).

3. Centrilobular emphysema causes structural changes of the central acinar respiratory bronchioles _____ (including, excluding) the distal lung units such as the alveolar ducts and alveoli.

ETIOLOGY

4. The two major contributing factors of emphysema are _____; and _____, a genetic disorder.

5. Cigarette smoke _____ (increases, decreases) protease activity that causes destruction of the lung parenchyma.

6. Cigarette smoke _____ (increases, decreases) the mucociliary function that leads to _____ (clearance, retention) of secretions.

Study the roles of α_1PI under normal and abnormal conditions as follows and answer questions 7 and 8.

Sequence of Events with Normal α_1PI Level

1. Normal integrity of lung tissues is maintained by elastin.
2. Elastin can be destroyed by elastase.
3. Elastase is kept in check by α_1PI.

Sequence of Events with α_1PI Deficiency

1. Deficiency of α_1PI
2. Excessive elastase level
3. Destruction of elastin
4. Destruction of lung tissues

7. Elastase is an enzyme released from a form of white blood cells (polymorphonuclear leukocytes) and macrophages. When the level of elastase is too high and left unchecked, it breaks down _____ _____, a substance that maintains the integrity of lung tissues.

8. α_1PI inhibits the actions of elastase, an enzyme that _____ (repairs, destroys) lung tissues. Deficiency of α_1PI _____ (increases, decreases) the activities of elastase, leading to destruction of elastin and eventually lung tissues. This condition commonly causes _____ (centrilobular, panlobular) emphysema.

PATHOPHYSIOLOGY

9. Emphysema causes destruction of lung tissue and loss of elastic recoil. Therefore, the expiratory flows are _____ (increased, decreased), driving pressure (breathing efficiency) is _____ (increased, decreased), compliance is _____ (increased, decreased), and elastance is _____ (increased, decreased).

10. Chronic air trapping and hyperinflation in emphysema are contributing factors that may lead to the reduction of a patient's _____ .
    A. functional residual capacity
    B. residual volume
    C. alveolar capillary beds and surface area for gas exchange
    D. total lung capacity

11. Which of the following is *least* likely a characteristic of emphysema? _____ _____ .
    A. $\dot{V}/\dot{Q}$ mismatch
    B. dead space ventilation
    C. increased work of breathing
    D. low lung compliance

CLINICAL FEATURES

12. The medical and personal history of emphysema may include all the following **EXCEPT:** _____ _____ .
    A. dyspnea at rest or on exertion
    B. signs of chronic bronchitis
    C. intrapulmonary shunting
    D. respiratory tract infection
    E. smoking history

13. On physical examination of a patient with emphysema, one may find all the following signs with the **EXCEPTION** of: _____ .
    A. use of accessory respiratory muscles
    B. prolonged inhalation phase
    C. barrel chest
    D. pursed-lip breathing on exhalation
    E. digital clubbing

14. To facilitate ventilation, patients with emphysema usually assume a sitting position while leaning _____ (forward, backward) supported by the elbows on a table.

15. The chest radiographs of emphysema usually show _____ (dome-shaped, flattened) hemidiaphragms, _____ (small and vertically, large and horizontally) oriented heart, and _____ (increased, decreased) retrosternal space.

16. The pulmonary function studies done on patients with emphysema may reveal _____ _____ (increase, decrease) in flow rates and _____ (increase, decrease) in residual volume, functional residual capacity, and total lung capacity. This condition is primarily due to chronic _____ (hypoxia, hyperventilation, air trapping).

17. In advanced and severe emphysema, arterial blood gases usually show hypoxemia with compensated or partially compensated respiratory _____ (acidosis, alkalosis).

18. Hyperinflation of the lungs and depression of the diaphragm make the heart assume a more _____ _____ (vertical, horizontal) position. It also causes a right shift of the _____ _____ (P, QRS, P and QRS) on the electrocardiogram tracings.

TREATMENT

19. Treatments for emphysema include pulmonary rehabilitation and oxygen therapy when the Pao_2 is less than _____ (55, 65, 75) mm Hg.

20. Acute care of emphysema patients should include all the following **EXCEPT:** _____ _____ .
    A. reduce the work of breathing
    B. perform complete pulmonary function studies
    C. provide adequate oxygenation
    D. use of bronchodilators
    E. improve ventilation

21. Smoke cessation, avoidance of respiratory infection and irritants, influenza vaccine, and proper nutritional support are all _____ (minor, important) parts of the overall treatment plan for emphysema patients.

22. Supplemental oxygen therapy should begin when the Pao_2 approaches _____ (40, 55, 70) mm Hg.

23. For airway obstruction, before- and after-_____ (steroid, antibiotic, diuretic, bronchodilator) pulmonary function studies should be done to select the most effective medication for home use.

24. Match the following types of medication with the appropriate use:

Medication	*Use*
A. steroid _____	1. improves ventilation
B. bronchodilator _____	2. clears infection
C. antibiotic _____	3. relieves fluid build-up
D. diuretic _____	4. reduces inflammatory response

25. Mechanical ventilation may be justified when the acute respiratory failure is caused by a(n) _____ (reversible, irreversible) problem superimposed on the chronic obstructive pulmonary disease (COPD) component.

26. In patients with $\alpha_1 PI$ deficiency, _____ (indomethacin, cromolyn sodium, Prolastin, albuterol) has been used with some short-term benefits.

CHAPTER **7**

CYSTIC FIBROSIS

1. Cystic fibrosis (CF) is an _____ (infectious, inherited) disease and its primary pulmonary involvement is characterized by _____ (croup, bronchiectasis, bronchitis).

2. CF primarily involves the following organs: _____ .
   A. lungs
   B. liver
   C. pancreas
   D. A and B
   E. A and C

ETIOLOGY

[**NOTES**: The autosomal recessive trait of CF is shown as follows: CC represents person afflicted with CF, CN represents person who carries the CF genes but is otherwise healthy, and NN represents normal person who does not carry the CF genes.]

PARENTS

CF + Carrier
(CC + CN)

	C	C
C	CC	CC
N	CN	CN

Carrier + Carrier
(CN + CN)

	C	N
C	CC	CN
N	CN	NN

CF + Normal
(CC + NN)

	C	C
N	CN	CN
N	CN	CN

EACH OFFSPRING'S CHANCES

50% (2/4) CF	25% (1/4) CF	100% (4/4) Carrier
50% (2/4) Carrier	50% (2/4) Carrier	
	25% (1/4) Normal	

3. CF is a genetic disorder and its inheritance pattern is an autosomal _____ (dominant, recessive) trait. Two carrier parents will have a _____ (25, 50, 75) percent chance of having a child with CF or without any trace of CF; a _____ (25, 50, 75) percent chance of having a child being a CF carrier.

PATHOLOGY AND PATHOPHYSIOLOGY

4. CF generally affects all exocrine glands. These exocrine abnormalities include all the following medical problems with the **EXCEPTION** of: _____ .
   A. chronic pulmonary infections
   B. renal failure
   C. exocrine pancreatic insufficiency
   D. elevated sweat chloride concentrations

5. In patients with progressive CF, the size of the pancreas is _____ (enlarged, diminished) and it has a(n) _____ (edematous, fibrotic) appearance. The pancreatic ducts and ductules are _____ (patent, obstructed) and the exocrine glands are eventually replaced with fibrous connective tissues.

6. Pulmonary involvement in CF includes all the following with the **EXCEPTION** of: _____
   _____ .
   A. pulmonary edema
   B. bronchiectasis
   C. frequent lung infections
   D. bronchial hyperactivity

7. In older patients with CF, their lungs become _____ (larger, smaller); the number and size of bronchial goblet cells are _____ (increased, decreased); mucus plugging is _____ (rare, common); and lymph nodes in the hilum of the lungs are _____ (enlarged, destroyed).

CLINICAL FEATURES

8. The medical history of a patient with CF usually reveals recurrent lung infections, digital clubbing, and dyspnea. In advanced stages, the patient may develop all the following signs **EXCEPT:** _____
   _____ .
   A. bronchiectasis
   B. hemoptysis
   C. pneumothorax
   D. epiglottitis
   E. cor pulmonale

9. _____ (Excessive, Deficiency of) pancreatic enzymes leads to maldigestion and poor absorption of food. Pancreatic exocrine insufficiency in CF is related to _____ (diarrhea, constipation) and _____ (fatty, bloody) stool.

10. Excessive sweat production causes a high concentration of _____ (salt, enzyme, macrophage) in sweat. Patients with CF _____ (do, do not) tolerate heat very well. They may also suffer from _____ (dehydration, overhydration) and electrolyte imbalance.

11. The upper respiratory symptoms of CF may include nasal polyps and recurrent _____
    _____ (cold, sinusitis, croup, epiglottitis).

12. CF patients are typically _____ (malnourished, well-nourished) children or young adults. They breathe with use of _____ (diaphragm, accessory muscles) and they often have _____ (productive, nonproductive) coughs.

13. Common physical signs of CF do **NOT** include _____ .
    A. decreased AP diameter of chest
    B. digital clubbing
    C. cyanosis
    D. cor pulmonale

14. In advanced stages of CF, jugular vein distension and pedal edema develop and they are caused by _____ (bronchiectasis, hypotension, cor pulmonale), also known as _____ (left, right)-sided heart failure.

15. The alveolar-arterial oxygen gradient in CF is usually _____ (increased, decreased) due to hypoxemia.

16. In the advanced stage of CF, arterial blood gases (ABGs) progress to severe _____ _____ (hyperoxemia, hypoxemia) and _____ (hypocapnia, hypercapnia).

17. The serum bicarbonate in ABGs is _____ (increased, decreased) because of renal compensation for chronic respiratory failure.

18. The hematocrit level in ABGs is _____ (increased, decreased) so that the oxygen-carrying capacity can be increased to compensate for chronic hypoxemia.

19. The chest radiograph of a patient with CF typically shows _____ (hypoventilation, hyperinflation), _____ (dome-shaped, flattened) hemidiaphragms, and a(n) _____ (increased, decreased) retrosternal space.

20. Because of severe airway obstruction, both the forced expiratory volume and forced vital capacity become _____ (increased, decreased) as the disease progresses.

21. Sweat chloride concentration of greater than _____ (20, 40, 60) mEq/L is required for confirmation of CF in _____ (children, adults). The concentration for _____ (children, adults) should be greater than 80 mEq/L to be diagnostic.

22. Common pathogens typically found in sputum of CF patients may include all the following **EXCEPT:**
    _____ .
    A. *Mycobacterium tuberculosis*
    B. *Staphylococcus aureus*
    C. *Pseudomonas aeruginosa*
    D. *Haemophilus influenzae*

TREATMENT

23. Heart or lung (or both) and bilateral lung transplants _____ (have, have not) been done successfully to treat end-stage CF.

24. To mobilize and expectorate the copious amount of respiratory secretions in CF, all the following modalities may be used with the **EXCEPTION** of: _____ .
    A. aerosolized deoxyribonuclease (DNase)
    B. postural drainage and chest physiotherapy
    C. voluntary coughing
    D. antibiotics
    E. positive expiratory mask

25. Repeated lung infections in CF are very _____ (common, unusual). Signs of respiratory infection in CF may include all the following **EXCEPT:** _____
    _____ .
    A. change in blood pressure
    B. change in cough and sputum characteristics
    C. fever
    D. deterioration in lung function
    E. lack of expected weight gain

26. Inhaled _____ (albuterol, gentamicin, DNase, Mucomyst) is commonly used to treat pulmonary _____ (edema, infection) in CF.

27. The treatment protocol for bronchial hyperactivity in CF should be the same as that for _____
    _____ (infection, hypertension, asthma, hypotension).

28. Pancreatic exocrine insufficiency in CF can best be managed with enzyme replacement and fat soluble vit-amins A, D, E, and K. (True or False) _____ .

29. Patients with CF should have a balanced diet consisting of high fat intake. (True or False) _____ .

PROGNOSIS

30. The prognosis for patients with CF has been _____ (improving, about the same) in recent years.

CHAPTER **8**

HEMODYNAMIC MONITORING AND SHOCK

INTRODUCTION

1. The circulatory system consists of all the following components **EXCEPT** the: _____
   _____ .
   A. pulmonary vasculature
   B. arteries and veins
   C. blood
   D. body tissue
   E. heart

2. Arteries carry blood _____ (to, away from) the heart and the veins carry blood
   _____ (to, away from) the heart.

3. A major structural or functional difference between veins and arteries is that _____
   _____ .
   A. veins have smooth muscle that can help regulate blood pressure
   B. arteries have smooth muscle that can help regulate blood pressure
   C. veins carry deoxygenated blood
   D. arteries carry oxygenated blood

4. Match each of the following functions with the respective organ that is responsible for the actions:

   Function

   A. controls muscle tone _____
   B. produces red blood cells _____
   C. gas exchange _____
   D. carries nutrients and waste _____
   E. processes nutrients _____

   Organ

   1. blood
   2. liver
   3. nervous system
   4. bone marrow
   5. lungs

5. The pulmonary _____ (veins, arteries) carry partially oxygenated or desaturated blood and the pulmonary _____ (veins, arteries) carry freshly oxygenated or saturated blood.

6. _____ (Pulmonary, Systemic) circulation is provided by the right ventricle and
   _____ (pulmonary, systemic) circulation is provided by the left ventricle.

7. Shock, or circulatory failure, may include all the following **EXCEPT:** _____
   _____ (hypertensive crisis, loss of sensorium, hypotension, renal failure, decreased urine output).

WHAT IS CARDIAC OUTPUT?

8. Cardiac output to the *systemic* circulation is the amount of blood that leaves the _____ (left, right) ventricle.

9. The normal cardiac output for an adult is about _____ (1 to 3, 2 to 4, 4 to 8) L/min.

10. The cardiac index (CI) is used to account for the variations in _____ (sex difference, body size). CI provides a representation of the cardiac output in relation to the size of the patient. It is determined by _____ (cardiac output and body weight, cardiac output and body surface area).

11. The average CI is about _____ (1 to 2, 2.5 to 4, 4 to 8) L/min/m².

WHAT DETERMINES CARDIAC OUTPUT?

12. Cardiac output is the product of stroke volume and _____ [cardiac output ($\dot{Q}$) = SV × ____].

13. Stimulation of the _____ (sympathetic, parasympathetic) nervous system causes the heart rate and cardiac output to increase under normal conditions. Conversely, bradycardia and decrease in cardiac output may result when the _____ (sympathetic, parasympathetic) nervous system is stimulated.

14. Stroke volume of the heart relies on the proper functions of all the following components **EXCEPT**:
_____ .
    A. cardiac index
    B. cardiac contractility
    C. ventricular filling volume (preload)
    D. arterial resistance to ventricular output (afterload)

Preload

15. Stretching of the myocardium by the venous pressure (venous return) during diastole is called _____ (cardiac contraction, preload, afterload).

16. Underfilling (i.e., hypovolemia) or overfilling (i.e., hypervolemia) of the ventricles causes a(n) _____ (increased, decreased) preload. In turn, the stroke volume is _____ (increased, decreased).

17. In reviewing a patient's chart for hemodynamic measurements on cardiac preloads, you would look up _____ (central venous pressure [CVP], pulmonary artery pressure [PAP], pulmonary capillary wedge pressure [PCWP]) for the right ventricular preload and the _____ (CVP, PAP, PCWP) for the left ventricular preload.

18. You are in the surgical intensive care unit monitoring a postoperative patient. The pulmonary artery (Swan-Ganz) catheter provides a CVP reading of 5 mm Hg and a PCWP of 12 mm Hg.

    Based on this information, you may conclude that the pressure readings are _____ _____ (lower than normal, higher than normal, within normal limits).

19. A patient with pulmonary edema is being monitored via a pulmonary artery (Swan-Ganz) catheter. The measurements are as follows: CVP = 13 mm Hg; PAP = 35 mm Hg; and PCWP = 20 mm Hg.

    Based on these measurements, you may conclude that the pressure readings are _____ _____ (lower than normal, higher than normal, within normal limits).

Afterload

20. The pressure created by the heart during contraction to overcome the arterial resistance is called the _____ (preload, afterload, filling pressure).

21. Systemic vascular resistance (SVR) is the arterial resistance of the systemic circulation. The circuit of resistance begins with the _____ measured by the _____ (mean arterial pressure, central venous pressure) and ends at _____ measured by the _____ (mean arterial pressure, central venous pressure).

22. Pulmonary vascular resistance (PVR) is the arterial resistance of the pulmonary circulation. The circuit of resistance begins at the _____ and is measured by the _____ _____ (pulmonary capillary wedge pressure, pulmonary artery pressure) ends at the _____ measured by the _____ (pulmonary capillary wedge pressure, pulmonary artery pressure).

23. Complete the following equations for calculation of SVR and PVR:
    SVR in dynes·s/cm^5 = _____ .
    PVR in dynes·s/cm^5 = _____ .

24. Adequacy of systemic circulation is partly dependent on the afterload of the left ventricle. Decreases in afterload (dilation of systemic vessels) will cause the blood pressure to _____ (rise, drop). If compensation is not forthcoming, the blood pressure may not be able to perfuse vital organs. This condition is called _____ (hypervolemia, shock).

Contractility

25. The ability and force of the heart to pump blood is called _____ (contractility, relaxation).

26. Optimal contractility, preload, and afterload are three requirements for normal _____ _____ (ventilation, cardiac output, metabolism).

27. When the cardiac contractility is decreased, the blood backs up in both the circulatory systems (pulmonary and systemic vascular systems). This causes the _____ (preload, afterload, preload and afterload) to increase.

28. *Negative* inotropes are factors that _____ (raise, reduce) the cardiac contractility. They include hypoxemia, acidosis, and β-adrenergic blockers.

29. *Positive* inotropes are factors that _____ (raise, reduce) the cardiac contractility. They include medications such as Isuprel (via stimulation of the sympathetic pathway) and atropine (via inhibition of parasympathetic pathway).

ETIOLOGY

30. Because normal cardiac output requires optimal contractility, preload, and afterload, inadequacy of any of these three functions can cause circulatory _____ (hyperperfusion, shock).

31. Match the cause of circulatory shock with its respective clinical example as follows:.

Cause of Circulatory Shock	*Clinical Example*
A. inadequate cardiac contractility _____	1. sepsis
B. inadequate preload _____	2. myocardial infarction
C. inadequate afterload _____	3. massive bleeding

32. Other causes of circulatory shock may include (1) massive pulmonary embolism in which the blood flow is greatly _____ (increased, obstructed); and (2) pericardial tamponade in which the cardiac contraction is _____ (excessive, inadequate).

33. Circulatory failure may be caused by septic shock, toxic shock, anaphylactic shock, or neurogenic shock. Among these different types of shocks, _____ is most common.

34. Septic shock affects the heart, vascular system, and other body organs and it is caused by toxins released by _____ (contaminated equipment, microorganisms).

PATHOPHYSIOLOGY

35. Match the system affected by shock with its respective clinical sign.

System Affected by Shock	*Clinical Sign*
A. brain _____	1. cool and clammy
B. kidneys _____	2. decreased urine output
C. peripheral circulation _____	3. decreased sensorium

36. Inadequate contractility of the _____ (left, right) ventricle can cause the blood to back up in the pulmonary circulation. If this condition is not corrected, it can lead to interstitial and pulmonary _____ (edema, fibrosis).

37. In severe shock where the lungs are underperfused, _____ (adult respiratory distress syndrome [ARDS], air trapping) can develop.

CLINICAL FEATURES

38. The common clinical signs of shock, regardless of cause, include all the following with the **EXCEPTION** of: _____ .
    A. tachycardia
    B. tachypnea
    C. hypotension
    D. weak peripheral pulse
    E. high blood pressure

39. Other clinical signs of shock include all the following **EXCEPT:** _____
_____ .

    A. diminished sensorium
    B. hypoxemia
    C. increased urine output
    D. cool and clammy skin
    E. shortness of breath

40. Severe shock often causes metabolic _____ (acidosis, alkalosis) due to tissue hypoxia, anaerobic metabolism, and accumulation of serum lactate (lactic acid).

41. In severe shock, the mixed venous oxygen tension ($P\bar{v}o_2$) can be _____ (higher, lower) than normal due to the continuing extraction of oxygen by the tissues in the presence of inadequate perfusion.

42. Significant electrolyte imbalance can affect the functions of the cardiovascular system. All the following are electrolytes **EXCEPT:** _____ (K^+, Na^+, $NaCl$, Cl^-, HCO_3^-).

43. Anion gap can be calculated by $Na^+–Cl^-–HCO_3^-$ and the normal range is between _____
_____ (–2 to 2, 2 to 6, 8 to 16) mEq/L. An anion gap higher than _____
_____ (2, 6, 16) may indicate the presence of lactic acidosis caused by severe shock and anaerobic metabolism.

    [NOTES: Metabolic acidosis with an *increased* anion gap is usually due to increased fixed acids resulting from renal failure, diabetic ketoacidosis, and *lactic* acidosis. These fixed acids may also be added to the body as in poisoning by salicylates and alcohols.

    Metabolic acidosis with a *normal* anion gap is usually caused by a loss of base. It is called hyperchloremic metabolic acidosis because this condition is usually related to accumulation of chloride ions.]

44. For patients with failure of vascular tone (e.g., septic shock, toxic shock), the body temperature can be _____ (higher, lower, higher or lower) than normal but the extremities remain warm and pink. The _____ (red, white) blood cell count is usually increased in this condition.

45. Patients who are at the peak of septic shock often present a(n) _____
(increased, decreased) cardiac output as a compensatory mechanism. A(n) _____
_____ (increased, decreased) systemic vascular resistance, and _____ (low to normal, normal to high) PCWP readings are also observed in these patients.

46. Late-stage septic shock syndrome causes depression of the myocardium. This in turn causes the cardiac output to _____ (increase, decrease).

47. Patients with hypovolemic shock usually show _____ (good, poor) perfusion to the extremities and therefore their _____ (warm, cool) digits have _____ (fast, slow) capillary refill. Peripheral cyanosis _____ (is, is not) commonly seen in hypovolemic shock.

48. On the electrocardiogram (ECG) tracings, _____ (tachycardia, bradycardia) is often seen in patients with hypovolemic shock. This is a compensatory mechanism for _____
_____ (excessive, inadequate) blood volume and cardiac output.

49. Changes (elevation or depression) in the ST segment or T-wave inversion on the ECG tracings may indicate that perfusion to the _____ (pulmonary, coronary, systemic) arteries is inadequate.

50. Use of vasopressors to correct _____ (hypertension, hypotension) should be done with great care because the compromised heart with an abnormal ST segment and T wave may not be able to tolerate an increased _____ (preload, afterload) from the vasopressor.

TREATMENT

51. Match each of the following primary treatments with the respective clinical condition:

    Treatment

    A. oxygen therapy _____
    B. endotracheal intubation _____
    C. PEEP _____
    D. mechanical ventilation _____

    Condition

    1. refractory hypoxemia
    2. respiratory failure
    3. hypoxemia
    4. prevent aspiration

    Refractory hypoxemia is present when the Pa_{O_2} is less than 60 mm Hg on an F_{IO_2} of 0.50 or greater.

52. In severe _____ (pump failure, septic, hypovolemic) shock, fluid replacement is the treatment of choice. The fluid should be properly matched blood. If matched blood is not readily available, volume expanders such as normal saline may be used to maintain adequate circulating volume.

53. Fluid replacement should be done when the systolic blood pressure is less than _____ (90, 110, 130) mm Hg and in most cases of hypovolemic shock. This is because hypovolemic shock lacks absolute circulating blood volume.

    [NOTES: (1) Fluid replacement should not be done in pump failure because excessive fluid can further stress the overworked heart. (2) Fluid replacement should not be used as the only or primary treatment for septic shock because reversal of septic shock can cause *hypervolemic* problems.]

54. Shock caused by pump (heart) failure requires careful diagnosis and proper treatment for the specific cardiac problem. Treatment for all kinds of shock _____ (does, does not) require close monitoring of the patient's hemodynamic status via a _____ (central venous, pulmonary artery) catheter.

55. Treatment of _____ (pump failure, hypovolemic, septic) shock includes antibiotics because this type of shock is caused by _____ (drug interactions, fluid depletion, microorganisms). Volume expanders may also be used to alleviate severe hypovolemia.

56. Vasopressors such as _____ or norepinephrine are useful to partially reverse the hypotensive crisis caused by septic shock.

CHAPTER **9**

PULMONARY THROMBOEMBOLIC DISEASE

INTRODUCTION

1. Besides fat deposits, there are many other materials that can produce embolism. They include all the following materials with the **EXCEPTION** of: _____ (air, blood serum, tumor fragments, amniotic fluid).

2. Pulmonary thromboembolism means obstruction of the pulmonary _____ (large airways, small airways, blood vessels) by blood clots. Blood clots are also called _____ _____ .

    [NOTES: Embolus is a mass of undissolved matter present in the blood or lymphatic vessel that may be solid, liquid, or gaseous. **Thrombus** refers to a blood clot that obstructs a blood vessel or a cavity of the heart.]

ETIOLOGY AND PATHOLOGY

3. List the *three* main causes for the formation of venous thrombi.

    _____

    _____

    _____

4. Genetic disorders in antithrombin III, protein S, protein C, and fibrinolytic abnormalities may result in the production of emboli because of the _____ .
    A. autoimmune disorders
    B. hypercoagulability factors
    C. hemolytic disorders
    D. hemophilia factor

5. A patient who was in a moving vehicle accident had surgery done to repair the femur. The medical history and clinical condition predispose the patient to the formation of emboli because of venostasis and

    _____ .
    A. hypercoagulability from loss of fibrin
    B. increased collateral venous blood flow
    C. damage to the venous blood vessels
    D. venous smooth muscle constriction

6. Prolonged immobilization from surgery or illness may promote the formation of emboli due to _____
_____ (slowed venous blood flow, increased prothrombin time).

7. List at least *five* other risk factors for the development of venous thrombosis.

_____

_____

_____

_____

_____

8. The most likely origins for venous thrombi are the _____
_____ .

    A. pulmonary veins
    B. brachiocephalic veins
    C. deep veins of the lower extremities
    D. deep arteries of the lower extremities

PATHOPHYSIOLOGY

9. Thromboemboli that obstruct pulmonary vascular perfusion usually leads to $\dot{V}/\dot{Q}$ mismatch in the form of
_____ (shunting, dead space ventilation). In this type of (high)
$\dot{V}/\dot{Q}$ mismatch, the pulmonary _____ (ventilation, perfusion) is much greater
than the _____ (ventilation, perfusion).

10. During a pulmonary embolism event, obstruction of pulmonary blood flow can also cause
_____ (increase, decrease) in surfactant production, _____
_____ (tension pneumothorax, atelectasis, consolidation) and hypoxemia. Bronchospasm may
also occur in pulmonary embolism.

11. Decrease in surfactant production is caused by the loss of pulmonary perfusion brought about by pulmonary embolism. It may cause all the following **EXCEPT:** _____
_____ .

    A. increase of lung compliance
    B. development of atelectasis
    C. formation of $\dot{V}/\dot{Q}$ mismatch
    D. progression of hypoxemia

12. During a pulmonary embolism event, the pulmonary vascular resistance (PVR) is normally elevated. This
is due to occlusion of the pulmonary blood vessels by the emboli and _____
_____ .

    A. vasoconstriction induced by hypoxia
    B. increase of lung compliance
    C. perfusion in excess of ventilation
    D. anticoagulation of the blood

13. In response to an increased PVR, the heart tries to overcome the PVR by _____
_____ .

    A. increasing the left ventricular function
    B. increasing the right ventricular function
    C. decreasing the left ventricular function
    D. decreasing the right ventricular function

14. If the right ventricle fails to provide an adequate blood volume, filling of the left ventricle _____ _____ (expands, diminishes) and _____ (hypertension, hypotension) results. Cardiovascular failure can occur because of severe systemic hypotension.

15. In healthy persons, systemic hypotension and cardiovascular compromise can occur when _____ (20, 50, 80) percent or more of the pulmonary vessels are occluded.

16. In patients with preexisting pulmonary or cardiovascular disease (e.g., chronic obstructive pulmonary disease [COPD], congestive heart failure (CHF), aortic or mitral valve disease), pulmonary hypertension usually has a _____ (greater, lesser) magnitude in a pulmonary embolism event. In these patients, systemic hypotension and cardiovascular compromise are usually more problematic than healthy individuals.

17. Fibrinolysis is the process of clot _____ (formation, destruction) and natural resolution of the thromboembolus begins _____ (shortly, long) after the clot lodges in the pulmonary blood vessels.

CLINICAL FEATURES

Medical History

18. Pulmonary embolism always occurs with very specific symptoms, and if risk factors are present, this makes diagnosis of pulmonary embolism definite. (True or False) _____ .

19. Acute _____ (angina pain, transient dyspnea) is the most common symptom associated with pulmonary embolism.

20. Other common symptoms related to pulmonary embolism include all the following with the **EXCEPTION** of: _____ .
    A. syncope
    B. pleuritic chest pain
    C. feeling of severe sickness
    D. hemoptysis
    E. systemic hypertension

21. Syncope is a transient loss of consciousness due to cerebral ischemia or _____ (excessive, inadequate) blood flow to the brain.

22. List *five* common *symptoms* of pulmonary thromboembolism.

    _____

    _____

    _____

    _____

    _____

Physical Examination

23. List *five* common *signs* of pulmonary thromboembolism.

    _____

    _____

    _____

    _____

    _____

24. On physical examination, patients with thromboembolism often show fever, tachypnea (respiratory rate _____ or greater), and tachycardia (heart rate _____ or greater).

25. Jugular vein distension may suggest _____ (left, right) heart strain causing backup of the venous blood flow.

26. Swelling and tenderness of the lower extremities may indicate deep _____ (arterial, venous) thrombosis.

27. On chest auscultation, localized wheezing or crackles may be heard. The breath sounds are _____ (sometimes, never) normal in patients with pulmonary thromboembolism.

28. A pleural friction rub may be heard if _____ (fluid, blood, infarction) is present involving the pleura.

29. Percussion of the chest wall usually shows _____ (pleural effusion, consolidation, normal findings).

30. On auscultation of the heart, loud P_2 sounds may be heard indicating sluggish or improper pulmonic valve _____ (opening, closure), which is caused by _____ (increased PVR, decreased pulmonary blood flow).

Hemodynamic and Laboratory Data

31. Monitoring with a pulmonary artery catheter may reveal the following hemodynamic changes in pulmonary thromboembolism (select one or more answer in each group):
    A. _____ (normal, high, low) central venous pressure

    B. _____ (normal, high, low) pulmonary artery pressure

    C. _____ (normal, high, low) pulmonary capillary wedge pressure (PCWP)

32. In pulmonary thromboembolism, a low PCWP reading can result from obstruction of the _____ _____ (systemic, pulmonary) blood vessels leading to _____ (excessive, inadequate) filling of the left heart.

33. The chest radiograph in pulmonary thromboembolism is usually normal with occasional pulmonary vascular distension due to _____ (high, low) blood pressure in the pulmonary circulation.

34. Arterial blood gases (ABGs) usually show uncompensated respiratory _____ (acidosis, alkalosis), _____ (mild to moderate, moderate to severe) hypoxemia, and a(n) _____ (increased, decreased) alveolar-to-arterial oxygen gradient ($P_{A}–a_{O_2}$).

35. Electrocardiogram (ECG) findings in pulmonary thromboembolism may show normal rhythm or sinus _____ (bradycardia, tachycardia) as a compensatory mechanism for reduced cardiac output. Premature ventricular contraction (PVC) is a(n) _____ (frequent, occasional, rare) finding.

36. A $\dot{V}/\dot{Q}$ scan is done to _____ .
    A. determine the cardiac output
    B. monitor systemic circulation
    C. rule out pulmonary embolism
    D. measure the $\dot{V}/\dot{Q}$ ratio

37. $\dot{V}/\dot{Q}$ scan using xenon-133 for _____ (ventilation, perfusion) and iodine-131 or technetium for _____ (ventilation, perfusion) often reveals _____ _____ (normal, increased, decreased) ventilation and _____ (normal, increased, decreased) perfusion in a patient with pulmonary embolism.

38. Pulmonary embolism can usually be confirmed when normal ventilation is associated with perfusion defects in _____ (one, two, three) or more lung segments or _____ (one, two, three) lobe(s).

39. Pulmonary _____ (function, angiography) is the most useful diagnostic test for pulmonary embolism but it has some associated complications making it the test of last resort.

TREATMENT

40. The initial treatment for pulmonary thromboembolism is _____ .
    A. surgical removal of the thrombi
    B. blood transfusion
    C. intravenous fluid
    D. intravenous heparin

41. Anticoagulant therapy is used to _____ (prevent the formation of new clots, dissolve the existing clots).

42. Thrombolytic therapy is done to _____ (prevent the formation of new clots, dissolve the existing clots). Agents used in thrombolytic therapy may include _____ _____ and _____ .
    A. warfarin (Coumadin) and streptokinase
    B. urokinase and streptokinase
    C. heparin and warfarin
    D. streptokinase and heparin

43. For patients with pulmonary embolism, the initial treatment for hypoxemia is _____ _____ (mask CPAP, high F_{IO_2}, mechanical ventilation). If respiratory failure develops due to severe pulmonary embolism, _____ (mask CPAP, IPPB, mechanical ventilation) would be indicated.

44. If hypotension develops during the pulmonary embolism event _____ may be used.
    I. vasodilator
    II. volume expanders
    III. dopamine
    IV. bronchodilator

    A. I only
    B. I and II only
    C. I, II, and III only
    D. II and III only
    E. all the above

45. All the following therapies are proved effective in the prevention of thromboembolism **EXCEPT:**
    _____ .
    A. low dose heparin
    B. early ambulation and use of elastic stockings
    C. sodium warfarin (Coumadin)
    D. venous compression devices

46. All the following are relative contraindications to thrombolytic therapy **EXCEPT:** _____
    _____ .
    A. recent surgery
    B. ulcers
    C. coronary artery disease
    D. cerebral vascular accident (stroke)

CHAPTER **10**

HEART FAILURE

1. Heart failure is diagnosed in approximately 400,000 people in the United States annually. The mortality rate in the first 2 years following diagnosis is about _____ percent of the total.
   A. 5
   B. 10
   C. 25
   D. 50

2. The mortality rate in heart failure is high because of _____ _____ .
   A. chronic pulmonary distress secondary to increased shunting
   B. renal insufficiency and associated hypernatremia
   C. hepatic shutdown secondary to hepatic hypertrophy
   D. multiple organ failure, perfusion loss, and stasis

3. Cor pulmonale is associated with _____ (right, left) heart enlargement and failure resulting from _____ (hypoperfusion, chronic pulmonary disease).

ETIOLOGY

4. Among the five leading factors, which of the following accounts for most cases of heart failure? _____ _____ .
   A. hypertension and coronary artery disease
   B. idiopathic dilated cardiomyopathy
   C. valvular abnormalities: regurgitation and stenosis
   D. congenital cardiac defects
   E. chronic pulmonary disease

5. Match the following conditions with the respective type of cor pulmonale (acute or chronic):

Conditions	Types
A. massive pulmonary embolism _____	1. acute
B. cystic fibrosis (CF) _____	2. chronic
C. emphysema _____	
D. adult respiratory distress syndrome (ARDS) _____	
E. abrupt rise of pulmonary artery pressure (PAP) _____	
F. chronic pulmonary hypertension _____	
G. severe hypoxic vasoconstriction _____	

PATHOPHYSIOLOGY

6. Cardiac output ($\dot{Q}_T$) is the _____ (sum, difference, product, dividend) of heart rate (HR) and stroke volume (SV).

7. Write the equation for $\dot{Q}_T$.

   _____

8. The pacing system of the heart directly determines the _____ (cardiac output, heart rate, stroke volume).

9. Venous return (preload pressure), downstream vascular resistance (afterload pressure), myocardial contractility, and ventricular compliance regulate the _____ (cardiac output, heart rate, stroke volume).

10. Congestive heart failure can be described as the inability of the heart to regulate _____ _____ (the pacing system, a balanced output).

11. The left heart has a _____ (thicker, thinner) myocardial wall and allows for a greater degree of compensation by _____ .
    A. sustaining a higher workload than the right heart
    B. sustaining a slower rate and using less oxygen
    C. varying preloads and afterloads
    D. having a larger reservoir than the right heart

12. In most cases, primary _____ (left, right) heart failure leads to failing of the other side. This is because the _____ (left, right) heart cannot withstand the drastic changes in preload and afterload as a result of _____ (left, right) heart failure.

13. Right heart failure seldomly leads to left heart failure because right heart failure _____ (increases, decreases) the blood flow and preload in the pulmonary circulation. Less pulmonary blood flow and a lower preload to the left heart act as a type of compensation for the left heart.

Myocardial Performance

14. The performance of the heart muscle fibers is dependent on its length-tension and force-velocity capabilities. Under normal conditions, the heart can pump out about _____ (20, 50, 70) percent of the ventricular blood volume in one heart beat. This is called ejection fraction.

15. End-diastolic ventricular volume is the blood volume in the _____ (atria, ventricles) at the end of diastole. Stroke volume is the blood volume pumped out of the ventricle in one _____ (minute, heart beat).

16. The ejection fraction is the amount of end-diastolic ventricular blood volume that _____ (is, is not) pumped from the heart by one heart beat (stroke volume). Normally it is about _____ (20, 50, 70) percent. In severe heart failure, the ejection fraction can be 20 percent or lower.

17. The ejection fraction can decrease under all the following conditions **EXCEPT:** _____
    _____ .
    A. decreased length-tension making contraction less efficient
    B. decreased force-velocity making blood flow inadequate
    C. stimulation of the β-receptors of the heart pacing system
    D. ventricular fibrillation
    E. cardiac arrest

18. One form of compensation for heart failure is the sympathetic response. In this form of compensation, an increase is noted in each of the following with the **EXCEPTION** of: _____ _____ .
    A. end-diastolic filling volumes
    B. contractility
    C. heart rate
    D. release of norepinephrine

19. In prolonged heart failure, continuing sympathetic compensation may challenge the ability of the _____ (endocardium, coronary arteries) to oxygenate the myocardium. Symptoms of ischemia may develop once the work of the heart exceeds the coronary arteries capacity to provide adequate blood flow.

20. Prolonged sympathetic compensation for heart failure may lead to a persistent _____ _____ (tachycardia, bradycardia) state that may be unresponsive to parasympathetic stimulation.

21. The Frank-Starling response describes the condition of myocardial contractility based on the relationship of stroke work and _____ (end-systolic, end-diastolic) volume.

22. Under normal conditions, an increase in venous return (preload) and ventricular filling (end-diastolic volume) causes the heart fibers to contract with _____ (greater, less) force.

    On the other hand, a decrease in venous return (preload) and ventricular filling (end-diastolic volume) causes the heart fibers to contract with _____ (greater, less) force.

23. In the event of heart failure, backup of blood flow causes a(n) _____ (increased, decreased) end-diastolic volume and ventricular _____ (dilation, contraction).

24. Excessive dilation (overstretching) of the ventricles to their upper limit causes the compliance of the heart to _____ (increase, decrease). This will _____ (augment, reduce) myocardial contractility and cardiac function.

25. Ventricular hypertrophy is usually a(n) _____ (chronic, acute) response to an increase of preload. This condition is characterized by _____ .
    I. increase of myocardial thickness
    II. increase of myocardial mass
    III. decrease of myocardial thickness
    IV. decrease of myocardial mass

    A. I and II only
    B. I and IV only
    C. II and III only
    D. III and IV only

26. Excessive ventricular hypertrophy causes the ventricular compliance to _____ (increase, decrease). This, in addition to ischemia caused by inadequate oxygen delivery, _____ _____ (increases, decreases) the work of the heart to compress the enlarged ventricles.

Peripheral and Pulmonary Circulation

27. To compensate for reduced cardiac output in heart failure, the systemic circulation diverts cardiac output to more vital organs _____ (from A to B, from B to A).
    A. renal and cutaneous tissues circulation
    B. coronary and cerebral circulation

28. In heart failure, the systemic vascular resistance is usually _____ (increased, decreased) due to the vasoactive effects of an elevated norepinephrine concentration and vasodilation from sodium and water absorption.

29. An increased systemic vascular resistance limits the blood flow, oxygen delivery, and heat dissipation. Therefore, patients with heart failure have very _____ (high, low) tolerance to heat and exertion.

Fluid and Electrolyte Balance

30. Reduced cardiac output and generalized vasoconstriction in heart failure can cause *arterial* _____ _____ (hyperperfusion, hypoperfusion) to the kidneys.

31. Backup of blood flow due to (right) heart failure can cause *venous* _____ (hyperperfusion, hypoperfusion) or congestion in the renal circulation.

32. Arterial hypoperfusion or venous hyperperfusion, or both in the renal circulation result in a reduced renal perfusion and glomerular filtration; and subsequently retention of sodium and water. (True or False) _____ .

33. In heart failure, renal insufficiency may be present because of _____ (increased, decreased) glomerular filtration rates.

34. _____ (Increased, Reduced) renal perfusion causes the kidneys to produce renin, which stimulates the production of _____ (angiotensin I, angiotensin II, angiotensin I and II).

35. Angiotensin I and II stimulate renal tubular sodium _____ (excretion, reabsorption) causing a _____ (high, low) level of sodium. The eventual vasoconstriction and renal hypoperfusion stimulate adrenal gland secretion of aldosterone, a chemical inducing further sodium _____ (excretion, retention).

36. As a result of these changes, patients with heart failure usually have increased blood volume, interstitial fluid volume, and total body sodium. In turn, fluid and electrolyte imbalance can lead to _____ _____ (pulmonary, systemic, pulmonary and systemic) edema.

Edema Formation

37. The movement of fluid between the blood vessels and interstitial space is mainly regulated by the permeability of the capillary wall and the balance between hydrostatic pressure and the osmotic pressure. Hydrostatic pressure (exerted by water in the capillary) tends to push the water *out of* the capillaries. Osmotic pressure (exerted by the protein concentration in the capillary) tends to draw the water *into* the capillaries.

    Under normal conditions, the _____ (inward, outward) driving force is slightly (10 mm Hg) higher, moving about 150 mL of fluid into the interstitial space per hour.

[**NOTES:** Pulmonary edema is usually caused by an increased hydrostatic pressure or an increased pulmonary capillary permeability. In high-pressure edema, the protein level in edema fluid is low. In high capillary permeability edema, the protein level in edema fluid is high.]

38. The 150 mL/hour of fluid in the interstitial space is absorbed by the _____ (pulmonary, cardiac, lymphatic) system and returned to the systemic venous circulation. When the fluid in the interstitial space builds up faster than the lymphatic system can handle, edema results.

39. In summary, edema is a clinical condition in which fluid accumulates in the _____ _____ (pleural, interstitial) spaces of the body. It may be caused by a(n) _____ _____ (increase, decrease) in capillary permeability, a(n) _____ (increase, decrease) in capillary blood pressure, a(n) _____ (increase, decrease) in blood protein concentration, and lymphatic obstruction.

40. The normal pulmonary capillary wedge pressure (PCWP) ranges from 6 to 12 mm Hg with a mean pressure of 8 mm Hg. In congestive heart failure, pulmonary edema is first noted when the PCWP exceeds _____ (6, 12, 18, 25) mm Hg. Clinical onset of edema occurs when the body retains and adds _____ (2, 3, 4, 5) liters of fluid.

Pulmonary Dysfunction

41. Mild pulmonary hypertension in the early stage of heart failure may have a desired effect on $(\dot{V}/\dot{Q})$ matching. This is because a higher pulmonary arterial pressure can _____ _____ .
    A. increase perfusion to poorly perfused areas
    B. increase ventilation to poorly ventilated areas
    C. decrease perfusion to overperfused areas
    D. decrease ventilation and perfusion

42. As heart failure advances, severe congestion in the pulmonary circulation and the resulting pulmonary edema can cause _____ .
    A. decrease in lung volumes
    B. decrease in airway resistance
    C. increase in diffusion capacity
    D. increase in gas exchange

43. In severe pulmonary edema, blood gases may show mixed respiratory and metabolic _____ _____ (acidosis, alkalosis). Respiratory acidosis is due to _____ (hyperventilation, hypoventilation) whereas metabolic acidosis is caused by prolonged hypoxia and _____ (aerobic, anaerobic) metabolism.

44. Match the severity of heart failure with the respective pathophysiologic change:

Heart failure	*Pathophysiologic Change*
A. mild _____	1. alveolar flooding
B. moderate _____	2. pulmonary vascular congestion
C. severe _____	3. pulmonary interstitial edema

CLINICAL FEATURES

45. In heart failure, the patient usually shows the following signs with the **EXCEPTION** of:
    A. shortness of breath
    B. generalized weakness
    C. delirium and incoherence
    D. reduced work of breathing

46. Peripheral pallor, digital cyanosis, and diaphoresis are some signs of heart failure due to _____ _____ (increase, reduction) of cardiac output and peripheral perfusion.

47. Heart failure creates backup of blood flow in the pulmonary and systemic circulations. When the pulmonary circulation is involved, pulmonary _____ (atelectasis, congestion) results. When the systemic circulation is involved, distended _____ (varicose, jugular, aqueous) vein and pitting edema of the ankles are common observations.

48. The accumulation of fluid in the interstitial space of the extremities to the point that pressure placed with the finger leaves a depression that takes several seconds to disappear is called _____ edema.

49. In interviewing a patient for recent medical history, the patient states that he or she needs several pillows during sleep to be able to breath. You would report this condition as _____ (Cheyne-Stokes breathing, dyspnea, tachypnea, orthopnea).

50. To compensate for the decreased cardiac output in heart failure, the heart rate is usually _____ (higher, lower) than normal. In addition, irregular heart beats may also be present.

51. Reduced cardiac output and arterial pressure causes the peripheral circulation and skin temperature to be _____ (raised, reduced).

52. On auscultation of patients with heart failure, _____ (crackles, wheezes, rhonchi) are heard when the air flow opens the collapsed lung regions. _____ (Crackles, Wheezes, Rhonchi) are heard when the airflow passes through airways that are narrowed or constricted.

53. Explain what causes airway narrowing in congestive heart failure.

    _____

    _____

54. Ms. Jones is admitted to the coronary unit with a diagnosis of chronic heart failure. The likely clinical features of this patient include _____ (large, small) liver and ascites or _____ (excessive, lack of) peritoneal fluid.

55. Hepatomegaly and ascites are caused by chronic venous _____ (hypertension, hypotension) and impaired lymphatic drainage. A clinical sign of this condition may be abdominal _____ (distension, depression).

Mild Failure

56. Mild heart failure is defined as pulmonary venous congestion with _____ (narrowed, widened) pulmonary arteries as seen on the chest radiograph.

Moderate Failure

57. In moderate heart failure, cardiomegaly, pulmonary engorgement, and presence of Kerley A, B lines are seen. Cardiomegaly is likely to have developed when the heart width (measured horizontally) is more than _____ (30, 50, 80) percent of the thorax width on the posterior-anterior (P-A) chest film.

58. Kerley A lines are the short (1 to 2 cm) lines of interstitial edema extending outward from the _____ _____ (hilum, pleural surface).

59. Kerley B lines are the short, thin streaks of interstitial edema outlining the lymphatics of a subsegmental region of lung that extends inward from the _____ (hilum, pleural surface).

Severe Failure

60. Which of the following features is **NOT** seen in severe heart failure? _____
_____ .
    A. cardiomegaly
    B. pulmonary artery engorgement
    C. PCWP of 18 mm Hg
    D. interstitial and pulmonary edema
    E. pleural effusion

61. Some of the electrocardiogram (ECG) abnormalities that may occur as a result of heart failure include all the following **EXCEPT:** _____ .
    A. ventricular fibrillation
    B. sinus tachycardia
    C. premature ventricular contractions
    D. atrial fibrillation
    E. bundle branch blocks
    F. ECG wave and segment changes

62. Arterial blood gases (ABGs) done on a patient with heart failure show an increased aveolar-arterial (A-a) gradient with the alveolar part remaining constant. The patient is dyspneic and has left ventricular hypertrophy. The recent radiographic study shows a butterfly pattern in the perihilar region. On auscultation, you hear inspiratory crackles and expiratory wheezes in all lung regions.

    If this patient develops pulmonary edema, it is most likely due to _____
    _____ .
    A. pulmonary artery hypotension
    B. elevation of PCWP to 15 mm Hg
    C. severe left heart failure
    D. tachycardia and atrial fibrillation

63. Respiratory impairment in heart failure is evident when the A-a difference in Pa_{O_2} becomes _____ (larger, smaller) and the Pa_{O_2} and FI_{O_2} are _____ (increased, reduced).

64. In prolonged heart failure and hypoxia, the patient becomes exhausted and the ABGs will show _____ (respiratory, metabolic) acidosis due to ventilatory failure and _____ (respiratory, metabolic) acidosis due to anaerobic metabolism under a hypoxic condition.

65. In chronic hypoxia due to heart failure, the hematocrit, hemoglobin, and erythrocyte levels are often increased. This change is a compensatory mechanism for increasing the _____ (oxygen, carbon dioxide, hydrogen ion) carrying capacity in the blood.

66. The serum sodium and potassium levels in patients with heart failure can be *low* if there is significant fluid retention or diuretic therapy. The normal range is 137 to 147 mEq/L for serum _____ (sodium, potassium) and 3.5 to 4.8 mEq/L for serum _____ (sodium, potassium).

67. Right heart failure causes systemic venous hypertension and eventual liver engorgement. When this happens, _____ (bilirubin, protease inhibitor, hematocrit) and liver enzyme levels will increase.

68. In heart failure, echocardiogram, Doppler flow, and radionuclide studies usually show significant _____ (improvement, impairment) in the functions of the heart.

69. Pulmonary artery catheterization is useful in gathering all the following data **EXCEPT:** _____
    _____ .
    A. cardiac output
    B. anatomic changes of the heart
    C. PAP
    D. left heart function

TREATMENT

Traditional treatment for heart failure is provided to manage the following *five* major areas of concern:
1. Reduce work of the heart (e.g., oxygen therapy)
2. Control sodium and fluid balance (e.g., fluid management)
3. Improve heart function (e.g., medications)
4. Prevent thromboembolism (e.g., heparin)
5. Support other organ functions (e.g., ventilation for lungs)

Management of Heart Failure

70. If heart failure causes an excessive afterload (due to backup of volume in the blood vessels), this problem can be managed by _____ (vasodilators, vasoconstrictors) such as direct-acting agents (e.g., nitroglycerine), indirect neurohumoral antagonistic drugs (e.g., captopril), and calcium channel blockers (e.g., verapamil). Other techniques to reduce an excessive afterload include appropriate physical and emotional conditioning, and sedation.

71. Sodium and water retention can be managed by use of a low _____ (calorie, fat, salt) diet and diuretics.

72. Drugs such as furosemide are used to reduce the work of the heart by
    A. correcting electrolyte imbalance
    B. preventing loss of body fluid
    C. improving cardiac contractility
    D. relieving pulmonary edema by diuresis

73. Diuretics should be titrated and given so as to obtain maximum cardiac output without causing pulmonary congestion. The target is a left ventricular preload (PCWP) of _____ mm Hg.
    A. 5 to 10
    B. 10 to 15
    C. 15 to 18
    D. 18 to 25

74. About _____ (2 hours, 1 day, 3 days) after reaching the ideal left ventricular preload pressure, crackles on auscultation and pulmonary edema on chest x-ray should clear.

75. Inotropic drugs such as dobutamine and digitalis are used to reduce the work of the heart by
    _____ .
    A. correcting electrolyte imbalance
    B. preventing loss of body fluid
    C. improving cardiac contractility
    D. relieving pulmonary edema by diuresis

76. A patient in the coronary care unit has been experiencing nausea, vomiting, sleeplessness, and disturbed color vision. You notice that he or she also has occasional arrhythmia on the cardiac monitor. To identify the cause of this condition, you would review the latest laboratory test on the _____ _____ .
    A. theophylline level
    B. carboxyhemoglobin level
    C. digitalis level
    D. bilirubin level

77. Frequent premature ventricular contractions (PVCs) seen in some heart failure patients may be due to excessive _____ (nitroglycerin, Versed, digitalis) level in the blood.

78. In heart failure patients, poor circulation may lead to the formation of emboli. Without the use of anticoagulant therapy these patients are at the greatest risk of developing pulmonary embolism and _____ _____ .
    A. dead space ventilation
    B. rapid venous stasis
    C. intrapulmonary shunting
    D. cardiac arrest

Respiratory Care for Cardiogenic Pulmonary Edema

79. Oxygen therapy and continuous positive airway pressure (CPAP) can be very effective for heart failure because it provides oxygenation by all the following mechanisms **EXCEPT:**
    A. decreasing the work of breathing
    B. improvement of gas exchange
    C. reduction of lung compliance
    D. reduction of pulmonary congestion

80. Respiratory failure with an increasing F_{IO_2} requirement of greater than 0.60 is an indication for _____ _____ .
    A. mask CPAP
    B. intubation and mechanical ventilation
    C. non-rebreathing mask
    D. drug therapy to stimulate respiration

81. You are managing a ventilator patient with a diagnosis of congestive heart failure with pulmonary edema. The serial blood gases show a normal and stable Pa_{CO_2} and a declining Pa_{O_2} (from 63 to 47 mm Hg) at an F_{IO_2} of 0.70. Which of the following would you suggest to the physician?
    A. initiate pressure support of 8 cm H_2O
    B. initiate positive end-expiratory pressure (PEEP) of 5 cm H_2O
    C. increase F_{IO_2} to 1.0
    D. increase tidal volume (V_T) by 100 cc

82. In the absence of obstructive lung disease, pulmonary edema may be managed by the following procedures **EXCEPT:** _____ .
    A. airway suctioning
    B. aerosolized bronchodilator
    C. diuretics

CHAPTER **11**

SMOKE INHALATION AND BURNS

INTRODUCTION

1. A vital piece of information you want to know when assessing a burn patient is whether there was smoke present in the fire. This is because smoke inhalation greatly increase the patient's _____ _____ .
    A. length of hospital stay
    B. functional residual capacity
    C. secondary infections
    D. mortality rate

2. The complexity of injuries sustained by a burn victim is due to all the following **EXCEPT:** _____ _____ .
    A. skin injury
    B. respiratory compromise
    C. sensory functions
    D. major organ system compromise

3. The management strategy to care for patients suffering from burn and smoke inhalation is grouped into _____ (two, three, four) overlapping phases.

4. Match the *three* phases of burn and smoke inhalation with the conditions and complications associated with each phase.
    A. early (resuscitative)
    B. intermediate (postresuscitative)
    C. late

Conditions and Complications

1. airway compromise _____
2. atelectasis _____
3. pulmonary edema _____
4. sepsis syndrome _____
5. pulmonary embolism _____
6. secretion retention _____

7. infectious pneumonia _____
8. hypermetabolic induced ventilatory failure _____
9. toxic gas inhalation _____
10. chronic pulmonary disease _____
11. adult respiratory distress syndrome (ARDS) _____

5. Fire-related morbidity and mortality rates are steadily declining due to all the following **EXCEPT:** _____ _____ .
    A. public education and awareness
    B. fewer house fires
    C. use of smoke detectors
    D. improved rescue techniques
    E. better established burn care

ETIOLOGY

6. The nature and extent of smoke inhalation injuries are influenced by the _____
   _____ .
   A. temperature of the fire and components of combustible materials
   B. location where victim was found and the victim's age
   C. both A and B

7. _____ (Air, Combustion) temperatures may reach 550°C (1022°F) or greater in 10 minutes or less if sufficient fuel is available.

8. In regard to steam production in a fire, steam produces _____ (10, 20, 500) times the heat energy that dry gases do at the same temperature.

9. Under the normal conditions in a fire, wood, cotton, and many acrylic materials produce aldehydes and organic acids. They are a source of _____ (carbon monoxide, respiratory irritants, smoke) in a fire.

10. During the course of a fire carbon dioxide (CO_2) levels may increase to _____ (1, 5, 10, 20) percent while oxygen (O_2) levels may decrease to _____ (1, 5, 10, 15) percent.

11. Carbon monoxide (CO) is produced in a fire due to _____ (complete, incomplete) combustion. Its level increases rapidly when the fire continues to burn in the _____
   _____ .
   A. presence of aldehydes and acrylics
   B. lack of oxygen
   C. lack of carbon dioxide
   D. presence of water vapor

12. Many toxic chemicals (carbon monoxide, hydrogen chloride, and phosgene) are produced by burning
   _____ .
   A. plastics containing polyvinyl chloride
   B. polyurethane materials such as nylon
   C. wood containing chemical treatments
   D. furniture containing fabric protectants

13. Hydrogen cyanide (HCN) and isocyanates are produced by burning _____
   _____ .
   A. furniture containing fabric protectants
   B. plastics containing polyvinyl chloride
   C. wood containing chemical treatments
   D. polyurethane materials such as nylon

14. Soot particles in a fire that are _____ (0.1 to 5, 5 to 10, 10 to 20) µm in size are carried into the lungs. Particles that are _____ (30, 50, 70) µm in size or greater are filtered out by the upper airways.

15. List *two* pathways in which chemical products in a fire can cause pathological changes to a burn victim.

   _____

   _____

PATHOPHYSIOLOGY

Early Pulmonary and Systemic Changes: 24 Hours Postburn

16. Exposure to the toxic and hypoxic environment of a fire disturbs oxygen transport and oxygen consumption. The condition affects the central nervous system and the _____ .
    A. kidneys
    B. integumentary system
    C. liver
    D. heart

17. Carbon monoxide has a very _____ (strong, weak) affinity for the oxygen-binding sites on the hemoglobin, thus making _____ (more, less) hemoglobin sites available for oxygen transport.

18. Carboxyhemoglobin (Hbco) concentration is measured in _____ .
    A. percent
    B. mm Hg
    C. vol%
    D. torr

19. Carboxyhemoglobin _____ (enhances, reduces) the transport and release of oxygen from hemoglobin by _____ (increasing, decreasing) the number of oxygen-binding sites on the hemoglobin.

20. In the presence of carbon monoxide (CO) poisoning a normal PaO_2 may not reflect the true cellular oxygenation status. (True or False) _____ .

21. Rapid cerebral edema may occur because of the following: _____ _____ .
    I. severe hypoventilation
    II. impaired oxygen transport
    III. increased carbon dioxide (CO_2) levels
    IV. hypotension

    A. I and II only
    B. I and IV only
    C. II and III only
    D. II and IV only

22. Lethal levels of CO poisoning are associated with a Hbco concentration that is greater than _____ (10, 30, 60) percent of the total hemoglobin level.

    [**NOTE:** The normal Hbco level in blood is less than 1 percent.]

23. Cyanide intoxication inhibits the cytochrome oxidase enzymes of the mitochondria. This has an effect of _____ .
    A. limiting the amount of hemoglobin
    B. increasing cellular respiration
    C. switching the tissues into anaerobic metabolism
    D. competing with the hemoglobin for oxygen binding sites

24. The principal causes of death in immediate-to-severe smoke inhalation are dysfunction of the cardiovascular and central nervous systems. These are the result of _____ .
    I. cellular anaerobic metabolism
    II. hypertensive crisis
    III. increase in dysfunctional hemoglobins
    IV. increasing carbon dioxide level

    A. I only
    B. I, II, and IV only
    C. I and III only
    D. I, III, and IV only

25. Thermal injury to the respiratory system includes the _____ .
    I. face and oral cavity
    II. nasal cavity
    III. pharynx
    IV. main-stem bronchi
    V. trachea

    A. I and II only
    B. I, II, and III only
    C. I, II, III, and IV only
    D. I, II, III, and V only

26. Thermal injury to the upper airways may occur within 2 to 8 hours. This can cause partial to complete closure of the glottis if the injury is severe. List *three* additional signs of upper airway injury.

    _____

    _____

    _____

27. The lower airways may be spared from thermal injury in some cases of smoke inhalation and burns. This is due to _____ .
    I. heat-induced pulmonary edema
    II. reflex laryngospasm
    III. glottic closure
    IV. cooling of the hot inspired gases by the upper airways
    V. mucus production

    A. I, II, and V only
    B. II, III, and IV only
    C. II, IV, and V only
    D. all the above

28. If the edema resulting from thermal injury of the upper airway progresses, ventilatory failure may occur as a result of _____ .
    A. loss of airway compliance
    B. loss of smooth muscle sympathetic response
    C. loss of a patent airway
    D. increased hypocapnia from tachypnea as a compensatory mechanism

29. In severe smoke inhalation, chemicals such as soot particles, irritating substances, and toxic gases can cause the following signs and symptoms: _____ .
    I. tracheobronchitis
    II. tracheoschisis
    III. bronchospasm
    IV. bronchorrhea
    V. pulmonary edema

    A. I, II, and IV
    B. I, III, and IV
    C. II, III, and IV
    D. I, III, IV, and V

30. The preceding changes caused by chemical injury may cause airway and alveolar edema. This is due to

    _____ .
    A. cellular changes secondary to the toxic events
    B. no vascular response resulting from loss of cardiac output
    C. increased bronchial blood flow
    D. loss of vascular tone

31. Other pulmonary abnormalities noted with chemical injury are surfactant dysfunction and (indicate whether the following will increase or decrease).
    A. lung water _____ (increase, decrease)
    B. lung compliance _____ (increase, decrease)
    C. pulmonary vascular resistance (PVR) _____ (increase, decrease)
    D. airway resistance _____ (increase, decrease)

32. The preceding conditions resulting from chemical injury can cause ventilation-perfusion ($\dot{V}/\dot{Q}$) mismatch. This will increase or decrease the following:
    A. $P(A–a)O_2$ gradient _____ (increase, decrease)
    B. V_D/V_T _____ (increase, decrease)
    C. minute volume _____ (increase, decrease)
    D. PaO_2 _____ (increase, decrease)

33. One of the early systemic changes caused by thermal injury is a substantial fluid shift _____ (to, from) the vascular system. This results in hypovolemia.

34. Within 8 to 24 hours post-thermal injury, the _____ of a burn patient reaches the highest point. The severity is dependent on the extent of the burn and the amount of fluid resuscitation.
    A. overall edema
    B. blood pressure
    C. infection
    D. respiratory impairment

35. Circumferential burns of the extremities and trunk may cause a(n) _____ (increased, decreased) skin compliance, skin elasticity, and chest wall compliance.

36. Circumferential burns of the extremities and trunk may affect the *respiratory* system by a(n) _____ _____ (increase, decrease) of the chest wall compliance, a(n) _____ _____ (increase, decrease) of the lung volumes, and development of _____ (respiratory alkalosis, ventilatory failure).

37. Circumferential burns of the extremities and trunk may affect the *circulatory* system by _____ _____ (increasing, decreasing) skin elasticity and compliance causing _____ _____ (increasing, decreasing) distal necrosis and edema.

38. The hemodynamic status of burn patients is usually compromised. The cardiac output is decreased due to suppression of cardiac functions and _____ (increased, decreased) in systemic vascular resistance.

Intermediate Pulmonary and Systemic Changes: 2 to 5 Days Postburn

39. During the 2 to 5 days postburn period, the patient exhibits _____ (increased, decreased) respiratory distress.

40. In the absence of pulmonary insult, a severely burned patient with stable lung functions may develop pulmonary edema. This edema may be caused by overly aggressive _____ (fluid, respiratory) therapy or _____ (increased, decreased) capillary permeability.

41. Burn patients usually begin to improve between days 2 and 4. If chemical injury persists, mucus production may be _____ (increased, decreased) and the function of mucus clearance may be _____ (enhanced, hindered).

42. Injuries to the _____ (trachea, bronchi, small airways) usually peak on day 2 or 3.

43. In more severe mucosal injuries, necrosis of mucosal tissues is common on day 3 or 4 postburn. This can lead to _____ (atelectasis, airway obstruction, atelectasis and airway obstruction)

44. Atelectasis may get worse because the patient's ability to breathe deep and cough is diminished due to a(n) _____ (increase, decrease) chest wall and lung compliance.

45. Reduced secretion clearance along with atelectasis and immune suppression place the patient at risk for _____ .

    A. respiratory failure
    B. leukocytopenia
    C. bacterial infections
    D. laryngotracheobroncholitis

46. ARDS is thought to be caused by a(n) _____ (increase, decrease) of surfactant production and a(n) _____ (increase, decrease) of pulmonary capillary membrane permeability.

47. During the 2 to 5 days postburn period, the patient's cardiac output is usually _____ (increased, decreased) along with the presence of _____ (tachycardia, bradycardia).

48. The patient's metabolic rate during this intermediate (2 to 5 days) phase is usually _____ (high, normal, low). This condition may last for 1 to 3 _____ (days, weeks, months).

Late Pulmonary and Systemic Changes: Beyond 5 Days Postburn

49. The primary cause of death in burn injury patients is _____ (pulmonary embolism, multiorgan failure), which is caused by _____ _____ (sepsis, surfactant depletion).

50. A(n) _____ (increased, normal, decreased) metabolic rate and CO_2 production continue during the late (beyond 5 days) postburn phase.

51. Increased work of breathing and eventual ventilatory failure may occur to burn patients in the late stage (beyond 5 days) due to persistent _____ (high, low) CO_2 production and muscle fatigue.

52. _____ (Pulmonary embolism, Pneumonia, Congestive heart failure) is a major problem for burn patients whether or not smoke inhalation is involved.

53. Pulmonary embolism occurs within 2 weeks postburn in 5 to 30 percent of burn patients. The diagnosis of pulmonary embolism may be confirmed by _____.
    I. chest x-ray
    II. serial $P(A\text{-}a)o_2$ studies
    III. pulmonary angiography
    IV. $\dot{V}/\dot{Q}$ scan
    V. $C(a\text{-}v)o_2$ studies

    A. I, II, and V
    B. I, IV, and V
    C. II and III
    D. III and IV

CLINICAL FEATURES

54. Exposure to asphyxiating conditions or carbon monoxide (CO) and cyanide (HCN) poisoning, or both, may lead to unconsciousness. CO poisoning can be determined by _____ (arterial blood gases [ABGs], pulse oximetry, co-oximetry).

55. Blood Hbco concentration of greater than _____ (5, 20, 60) percent may cause coma, shock, apnea, or death.

56. The use of pulse oximetry is a quick and noninvasive diagnostic tool for assessment of the oxygenation status of a patient. In the presence of dysfunctional hemoglobin such as Hbco, pulse oximetry will report a(n) _____ .
    A. accurate Hbo_2 value
    B. lower than actual O_2 saturation value
    C. higher than actual O_2 saturation value
    D. accurate Po_2 value

57. On examining a burn patient, you notice the following signs: singed nasal hair, facial burns, carbonaceous deposits in the upper airway, and oral and laryngeal edema. These signs _____ (suggest, conclude) that inhalation injury has occurred to the patient.

58. On further examination of the burn patient in the preceding question, you observe chest retraction in addition to audible hoarseness, dysphonia, and stridor. These signs suggest _____ (upper airway, lung parenchymal, septic) injury.

59. In addition to the signs of a burn patient in the two preceding questions, cough, cyanosis, wheezing, rhonchi, crackles, or dyspnea indicate that a _____ (more, less) severe inhalation injury has occurred.

60. Chest radiograph _____ (often, rarely) shows small airway injury due to smoke inhalation.

61. Patients with inhalation injury may have small and upper airway changes. To assess these changes _____ _____ (peak flow, forced expiratory flow during the middle half of the forced vital capacity [$FEF_{25-75\%}$]) is useful in assessing small airway changes whereas _____ _____ (peak flow, $FEF_{25-75\%}$) is useful in the assessment of upper airway changes.

62. ABG gas samples may be used to track the progress of the patient's condition. The $P(A-a)O_2$ that is (greater than, less than) _____ 300 mm Hg or a Pao_2/Fio_2 that is (greater than, less than) _____ 350 mm Hg are indicative of impaired pulmonary function.

63. A common finding in the early postburn state is respiratory _____ (alkalosis, acidosis), which is a compensatory mechanism for the hypermetabolic rate. In the presence of ventilatory failure and severe hypoxemia, respiratory _____ (acidosis, alkalosis) is usually found.

64. Evaluation of cutaneous damage is achieved by the _____ .
    A. Dubowitz index
    B. rule of nines
    C. appearance of the skin
    D. Silverman-Anderson burn scale

65. Assign the degree of burn (first, second, or third) to the following signs of burn depth and characteristics:
    A. _____ degree burn extends to the dermis with erythema, blisters, and pain
    B. _____ degree burn extends to the epithelium with erythema and pain
    C. _____ degree burn may extend to the hypodermis with pale or brown leathery skin, and no pain

TREATMENT

66. List *seven* goals of respiratory care for the burn patient.

_____

_____

_____

_____

_____

_____

_____

67. Supplemental oxygen may be delivered by nasal cannula, and a high Fowler's position (45 to 60 degrees) may be used to assist in ventilation because this position tends to reduce the patient's _____.
    A. lung compliance
    B. chest wall compliance
    C. functional residual capacity
    D. work of breathing

68. Bronchospasm may be treated by using a(n) _____ (vasoconstrictor, antibiotic, bronchodilator, β-antagonist).

69. If upper airway obstruction is expected, an endotracheal tube may be used. Early tracheostomy is usually _____.
    A. preferred in most cases to prevent trachea trauma from the endotracheal tube
    B. preferred for short-term ventilatory support because pulmonary hygiene is easily accomplished
    C. not preferred because of infections and high mortality rates
    D. not preferred because burn patients require only short-term ventilatory support

70. Use of continuous positive airway pressure (CPAP) may decrease early mortality rate in burn patients. List *four* additional reasons for using 5 to 10 cm H_2O of CPAP for these patients.

    _____

    _____

    _____

    _____

71. Patients with less than 30 percent Hbco and stable cardiopulmonary functions should _____.
    A. have blood gases every 24 hours until Hbco levels are less than 2 percent
    B. receive 4 liters of oxygen per cannula until Hbco levels are less than 5 percent
    C. receive 100 percent oxygen via non-rebreathing mask until Hbco levels are less than 10 percent
    D. use a partial-rebreathing mask until Hbco levels are less than 5 percent

72. Patients with increasing hypoxemia and little or no thermal injury to the face and upper airways may benefit from _____.
    A. heated aerosol with 100 percent FIO_2
    B. mask CPAP with 100 percent FIO_2
    C. intermittent positive pressure breathing (IPPB) treatments with bronchodilator
    D. nasal CPAP with 100 percent FIO_2

73. Burn patients who require intubation and mechanical ventilation usually have all the following contributing factors **EXCEPT:** _____.
    A. coma
    B. refractory hypoxemia
    C. inhalation injury
    D. cardiopulmonary instability
    E. respiratory alkalosis

74. Hyperbaric oxygen therapy may be beneficial to the burn patient by improving oxygen transport and _____.
    A. decreasing dead space ventilation
    B. increasing lung volumes
    C. increasing the removal rate for Hbco
    D. maintaining patent airways

75. Burn patients who have severe respiratory _____ (acidosis, alkalosis) and _____ (hypoxemia, hyperoxemia) often require ventilatory support. In addition, positive end-expiratory pressure (PEEP) is indicated when the Pa_{O_2} falls below 60 mm Hg on an F_{IO_2} of _____ (25, 40, 60) percent or greater.

76. Pulmonary hygiene such as chest physical therapy and therapeutic fiberoptic bronchoscopy can be helpful to mobilize secretions or to help prevent atelectasis and _____ (airway plugging, pulmonary edema).

77. To prevent renal failure, shock, and pulmonary edema fluid maintenance is vital. The ideal goals in fluid maintenance are a urine output of _____ (5 to 10, 30 to 50) mL/hour and a central venous pressure (CVP) reading of _____ (2 to 6, 8 to 12) mm Hg.

78. Large caloric intake (up to 150 percent of resting requirement) is necessary for patients who have extensive burns because it _____ (promotes, prevents) the catabolic process and enhances the healing of skin.

79. Escharotomy (cutting of burned skin) of the burned chest wall will directly improve the chest wall _____ and relieve the _____ (compressive, expanding) effect of retracting scar tissues.

80. In addition to débridement of dead skin, list *three* other conventional methods of burn wound treatment.

_____

_____

_____

81. All the following factors play a role in the prevention of infection in burn patients with the **EXCEPTION** of: _____ .
    A. cultures from body fluids and wound site
    B. room pressurization
    C. prophylactic corticosteriods
    D. air filtration
    E. wound covering

CHAPTER **12**

NEAR DROWNING

INTRODUCTION

1. Death caused by suffocation resulting from submersion is called drowning. Fluid is aspirated in _____ (10 to 15, 85 to 90) percent of the cases. Asphyxia from acute laryngospasm or prolonged breath holding claims _____ (10 to 15, 85 to 90) percent of all drowning victims.

2. A near-drowning victim is one who has been successfully resuscitated _____ _____ .
   A. and survives for at least 48 hours
   B. and survives for at least 24 hours
   C. at the scene and requires no hospitalization
   D. at the scene and requires hospitalization for observation

3. About half of all teenage drownings are related to the use of _____ (alcohol, drugs, life vests).

PATHOLOGY AND PATHOPHYSIOLOGY

Neurological Insult

4. _____ (Hypoxia, Ischemia) means an insufficient oxygen supply to a particular tissue of the body.

5. _____ (Hypoxia, Ischemia) means an insufficient blood supply to a particular tissue of the body.

6. A diminished blood supply will decrease oxygen transport. Loss of consciousness occurs to most people after _____ (2, 4 to 6, 8 to 10) minutes of anoxia. Brain damage may occur within _____ (2, 4 to 6, 8 to 10) minutes.

   [NOTES: Normal oxygen consumption is about 250 mL/min while breathing room air. The body's available oxygen stores are about 450 mL of O_2 in the lungs and about 500 mL of O_2 in the blood. Therefore, almost 50 percent of all oxygen available is depleted in just 2 minutes].

7. Full recovery in near-drowning victims has been seen after prolonged submersion in cold water for as long as 40 minutes. This extraordinary outcome is probably due to the diving reflex that includes breath holding, _____ (bradycardia, tachycardia), and peripheral _____ _____ (vasodilation, vasoconstriction). In addition to the diving reflex, the brain-protective effects (a reduced metabolic demand in the presence of extreme low body temperature) also contribute to this outcome.

8. List the *three* major metabolic pathways that produce adenosine triphosphate (ATP).

_____

_____

_____

Study the following sequence and then anwer question 9:

Sequence of Events Caused by Anaerobic Metabolism

1. ATP production is decreased to 2 ATP (from 36 ATP in aerobic metabolism)
2. Oxygen and energy supply is decreased
3. Cellular integrity is compromised
4. K^+ readily moves outside of cells
5. Na^+ and Ca^{2+} move into cells to maintain electroneutrality
6. Water follows Na^+ and Ca^{2+} causing swelling of cells
7. Lactate (lactic acid) is produced causing metabolic acidosis

9. Under anaerobic conditions the production of ATP is limited to one pathway in which _____ _____ .
   A. tricarboxylic acid cycle produces a net of 2 ATP compared with 36 under aerobic conditions
   B. oxidative phosphorylation produces a net of 2 ATP compared with 36 under aerobic conditions
   C. Krebs cycle produces a net of 2 ATP compared with 36 under aerobic conditions
   D. glycolysis produces a net of 2 ATP compared with 36 under aerobic conditions

10. Brain cells require an aerobic condition to carry on normal cellular activity. What would be the end result when the brain cells metabolize in an anaerobic environment? _____ .
    A. electrolyte imbalance
    B. cellular distension
    C. cellular collapse
    D. severe alkalosis

Pulmonary Insult

11. The degree of pulmonary damage inflicted by a near-drowning event is determined by _____ _____ .
    A. amount and type of aspirated fluid
    B. length of time under water
    C. length of time before effective cardiopulmonary resuscitation (CPR) is initiated
    D. volume, type, and components of the aspirate

12. _____ (Salt water, Freshwater) is a hypotonic solution when compared with blood. Once aspirated, it rapidly _____ (draws fluid from, enters) the pulmonary circulation. This abnormal condition in the lungs lowers the surfactant level and induces alveolar _____ (collapse, swelling).

13. _____ (Salt water, Freshwater) is a hypertonic solution when compared with blood. Once aspirated, it rapidly _____ (draws fluid from, enters) the pulmonary circulation. This abnormal condition in the lungs causes wash out of surfactant and induces alveolar _____ (collapse, swelling).

14. The resultant atelectasis may lead to refractory hypoxemia as well as _____ _____ .

    I. V̇/Q̇ mismatching
    II. increased thoracic compliance
    III. intrapulmonary shunting
    IV. decreased lung compliance
    V. diminished functional residual capacity (FRC)

    A. I, II, and III
    B. I, II, IV, and V
    C. I, II, and V
    D. I, III, IV, and V
    E. II, III, IV, and V

15. Near-drowning victims are prone to vomiting and aspiration, any aspirated substance may invoke an _____ (immunosuppresing, inflammatory) response in the entire respiratory tract. All the following conditions may occur **EXCEPT:** _____ .
    A. pleural effusion
    B. alveolitis
    C. bronchitis
    D. pneumonitis

16. A common complication of near drowning is _____ . This is a result of the inflammatory process and injury to the microvasculature of the lungs.
    A. pulmonary embolus
    B. noncardiogenic pulmonary edema
    C. pneumolysis
    D. pneumoconiosis

Hemodynamic and Electrolyte Effects

17. Match the following clinical parameters with the type of changes you expect to see in near-drowning patients (you may use any answer more than once):

    Type of Change

    A. increase _____
    B. decrease _____
    C. no change _____

    Hemodynamic, Electrolyte, and Blood Parameters

    1. dynamic compliance
    2. pulmonary capillary wedge pressure (PCWP)
    3. hemoglobin and hematocrit (salt water near drowning)
    4. hemoglobin and hematocrit (freshwater near drowning)
    5. central venous pressure (CVP)
    6. cardiac output
    7. electrolytes
    8. pulmonary vascular resistance (PVR)

    [NOTES: Hemoglobin, hematocrit, and electrolyte concentrations may decrease when *large* volumes of *freshwater* are swallowed or aspirated. This is due to dilution of the circulating blood volume by water.]

18. _____ (Hypoxia, Hypercapnia, Aspiration of fluid) is believed to cause the initial changes in the cardiovascular and hemodynamic function of a near-drowning patient.

Renal Function

19. Renal function is not usually impaired from near drowning. However, _____ (azotemic renal failure, acute tubular necrosis) may occur when renal hypoperfusion, lactic acid production, trauma, or *myoglobinuria* is present.

Myoglobinuria is myoglobin in the urine. It may occur as a result of muscular activity or trauma, or as a result of a deficiency of muscle phosphorylase (an enzyme that catalyzes the formation of glucose-1-phosphate from glycogen).

CLINICAL FEATURES

20. Assessment of near-drowning victims is critical and should be focused on the level of consciousness, pulse, and respiratory rate. List *eight* other sources of information that would be useful for resuscitation and postresuscitation care.

_____

_____

_____

_____

_____

_____

_____

_____

21. The vital signs (pulse, respiration, temperature, and blood pressure) of a near-drowning victim are highly variable. Factors that can influence the body temperature of a patient include all the following **EXCEPT:** _____ .

A. water temperature
B. duration of submersion
C. patient's P_{O_2} level
D. patient's body surface area

22. Cardiac involvement in a near-drowning victim usually results in _____ (tachycardia, bradycardia) possibly followed by _____ (asystole, ventricular fibrillation).

23. Neurological damage from hypoxia and rescue drugs will result in _____ (dilated, constricted) pupils that are _____ (fast, slow, slow to nonreactive) to light.

24. Match the following breath sounds with the associated clinical conditions:

Breath sound

A. coarse crackles _____
B. wheezes _____
C. late inspiratory crackles _____

Condition

1. bronchospasm or foreign body aspiration
2. atelectasis or pulmonary edema
3. aspiration of fluid

25. Because most near-drowning victims suffer from hypothermia and peripheral vasoconstriction, their extremities may show slow capillary refill and _____ .
A. central cyanosis
B. erythema
C. petechiae
D. skin that is cool to the touch

26. For near-drowning patients, hypoxemia and _____ are two common findings in arterial blood gas (ABG) reports.
    A. metabolic alkalosis
    B. metabolic acidosis
    C. respiratory alkalosis
    D. combined alkalosis

27. Hemoglobin, hematocrit, and electrolyte levels may decrease if large volumes of _____ (freshwater, salt water) are swallowed or aspirated.

INITIAL ASSESSMENT AND PROGNOSIS

28. Assessment of the near-drowning victim may be done by all the following **EXCEPT** the: _____ _____ .
    A. Silverman-Anderson scale
    B. postsubmersion neurological classification system
    C. Orlowski score
    D. Glasgow coma scale

Use the following information to anwer question 29:

GLASGOW COMA SCALE

Signs	Points and Responses
eye opening	1. none 2. to pain 3. to speech 4. spontaneous
best verbal response	1. none 2. incomprehensible 3. innappropriate 4. confused 5. oriented
best motor response	1. none 2. extension (decerebrate) 3. flexion (decorticate) 4. localizing pain 5. obeying commands

Decerebrate: Removal of the brain or cutting the spinal cord at the level of the brain stem. The patient's extremities are stiff and extended, and the head is retracted.

Decorticate: Lesion at or above the upper brain stem. The patient is rigidly still with arms flexed, fists clenched, and legs extended.

29. Based on the Glasgow coma scale, what total score indicates the presence of a coma?

_____

30. You are a respiratory therapist assigned to the emergency department. One hour into your shift you are paged and asked by the physician to assess an 8-year-old near-drowning patient. Assessment using the Glasgow coma scale reveals the following:
    A. answers to simple questions incomprehensible
    B. eyes open on pain stimulation
    C. arms rigid and flexed

    Based on your assessment, the individual scores are _____ , _____ , and _____ , respectively; and the total score is _____ . This total score indicates _____ (presence, absence) of coma.

31. In assessing a near-drowning victim, what are the *five* unfavorable prognostic factors in the Orlowski score?

    _____

    _____

    _____

    _____

    _____

32. The physician asks you to gather further information on the near-drowning event. You would interview the witnesses to the near drowning and use the Orlowski scoring system for your assessment. Your interview reveals the following:
    A. 8-year-old patient submerged in water for about 2 minutes
    B. trained medical personnel present and began CPR immediately
    C. ABGs on admission, pH 7.10, Pao_2 = 42 mm Hg, $Paco_2$ = 78 mm Hg
    D. patient unconscious on arrival to the emergency department

    Based on the results of this interview, there is (are) _____ (1, 2, 3, 4) unfavorable factor(s) based on the Orlowski scoring system. Therefore, the prognosis for this patient is quite _____ (good, poor).

33. It is 4 hours following resuscitation and the family physician asks you to review the patient's admitting condition using a postsubmersion neurological classification system. Based on the information obtained from the last question, you would report to the physician that the patient is in a _____ _____ state.
    A. category A
    B. category B
    C. category C

TREATMENT

34. In treating a near-drowning victim, basic cardiac life support (BCLS) and activation of the emergency medical services (EMS) should be done as soon as possible. Assessment for a pulse should be done when the patient is _____ (in the water, out of the water).

35. The Heimlich maneuver _____ (should, should not) be done to a near-drowning victim unless the airway is obstructed.

Category A (Awake)

36. Based on the postsubmersion neurological classification system, patients in category A have minimal neurological injury and exhibit which of the following? _____ .
    I. alert and awake
    II. a Glasgow coma scale of 9 to 11
    III. arousable but lethargic
    IV. a Glasgow coma scale of 14
    V. spontaneous eye opening, with confused responses

    A. I and II
    B. I and IV
    C. I and V
    D. II and V
    E. III and IV

37. In addition to complete blood count (CBC), electrolytes, chest radiograph, ABGs, sputum cultures, glucose levels, and clotting times, cervical radiograph should be done to rule out _____ _____ (congenital spina bifida, head injury, neck fracture).

38. Treatment for this group of patients is primarily symptomatic. Oxygen is used to keep Po_2 above _____ (40, 60, 80) mm Hg. Foreign body aspiration may be assessed by _____ _____ (pulmonary function test, chest x-ray). _____ (Antibiotics, Bronchodilators) may be used for bronchospasm. Fluid and electrolyte balance may be maintained, if necessary, by inserting an _____ (intra-arterial, intravenous) line.

39. In near-drowning patients, neurological deterioration may occur with all the following factors **EXCEPT:**
    _____ .
    A. hypocapnia
    B. hypoxemia
    C. deteriorating pulmonary function
    D. drug use before the near-drowning event
    E. increasing intracranial pressure

Category B (Blunted)

40. Based on the postsubmersion neurological classification system, patients in category B have moderate neurological injury and they usually show all the following signs **EXCEPT:** _____
    _____ .
    A. Glasgow coma score of 10 to 13
    B. irritable and combative
    C. prolonged periods of asphyxia
    D. obtunded (dull) but arousable
    E. dilated pupils and nonreactive to light

41. Category B patients _____ (should, should not) have all laboratory work for category A patients. Blood, sputum, and urine cultures should be done to evaluate the need for _____ (blood transfusion, fluid administration, antibiotics).

42. Which of the following vitamins may be used to improve the clotting times? _____
    _____ .
    A. vitamin A
    B. vitamin B
    C. vitamin C
    D. vitamin D
    E. vitamin K

43. Antibiotics should be used in near-drowning patients _____ (as a prophylactic measure, when culture results are positive).

44. Fluid management can be monitored by keeping the serum osmolarity level at or below _____ (280, 320, 360) _____ (mEq/L, mOsm/L).

Category C (Comatose)

45. Based on the postsubmersion neurological classification system, patients in category C have severe neurological injury. They are usually not arousable and their Glasgow coma score is less than _____ (3, 7, 10).

46. List *six* areas of treatment that must be maintained for near-drowning patients.

_____

_____

_____

_____

_____

_____

47. Diuretics are used to control _____ (atelectasis, pulmonary edema) and to prevent an increasing _____ (intracranial pressure, peak airway pressure).

48. Monitoring of hemodynamic values is done to prevent excessive _____ _____ (hydration by fluid infusion, dehydration by fluid restriction) that may lead to renal insufficiency and failure.

49. Near-drowning patients should be hyperventilated because hyperventilation _____ (increases, decreases) the pH. In turn, cerebral blood vessels respond to this pH by _____ (vasodilating, vasoconstricting), which can _____ (increase, decrease) the intracranial pressure.

50. A target $Paco_2$ of _____ (10 to 25, 25 to 30, 30 to 40, 40 to 50) mm Hg is desired when attempting to hyperventilate near-drowning patients.

51. List *two* common methods to hyperventilate a patient who is on the ventilator.

_____

_____

52. To maintain a Pao_2 of 60 mm Hg or higher, positive end-respiratory pressure (PEEP) may be necessary when _____ (dead space ventilation, intrapulmonary shunting) is present. PEEP should be raised in increments of _____ (5, 10, 15) cm H_2O for adult patients. For younger patients the increments should be _____ (larger, smaller, the same).

53. Induced hypothermia is not advised for treating near-drowning patients who are comatose and have suffered neurological damage. Induced hypothermia postbrain injury may lead to all the following changes **EXCEPT:** _____ .
    A. left shift of the oxyhemoglobin dissociation curve
    B. hypermetabolic rate
    C. cardiac dysrhythmias
    D. suppression of the immune system

54. Normothermia (normal temperature) may be achieved by the use of cooling mattresses and antipyretic (fever-reducing) agents. Correction of hyperthermia can help to reduce _____ .
    A. infection rate
    B. oxygen consumption
    C. expiratory flow rate
    D. fluid retention

55. Barbiturates are used to control _____ in the category C near-drowning patient.
    A. dehydration
    B. electrolyte balance
    C. enzymatic activities
    D. seizures

56. In treating the category C near-drowning patients, use of steroids _____

    _____ .
    A. is recommended to prevent the spread of infections
    B. is mandatory for control of infections
    C. may suppress the immune response and cause a higher incidence of infection
    D. has proved successful in controlling the intracranial pressure

57. Decerebrate and decorticate rigid posturing are signs of _____
    (raised, lowered) intracranial pressure (ICP). This condition may be caused by all the following **EXCEPT:**

    _____ .
    A. barbiturate use
    B. mechanical ventilation and PEEP
    C. hypoxia
    D. coughing
    E. prolonged suctioning

    Decerebrate: Complete absence of nerve impulse from the upper brain stem. The patient's extremities are stiff and extended, and the head is retracted. **Decorticate:** Lesion at or above the upper brain stem. The patient is rigidly still with arms flexed, fists clenched, and legs extended.

58. The intracranial pressure may be reduced by using any of the following **EXCEPT:** _____

    _____ .
    A. paralyzing agents
    B. induced hyperventilation
    C. sedatives
    D. pressure controlled ventilation

CHAPTER **13**

ADULT RESPIRATORY DISTRESS SYNDROME

INTRODUCTION

1. Adult respiratory distress syndrome (ARDS) is characterized by severe hypoxemia and respiratory _____ (alkalosis, insufficiency, failure) due to damage to the _____ _____ (pulmonary capillary, alveolar wall, alveolar-capillary membrane). This type of damage greatly _____ (increases, decreases) the permeability of the pulmonary vessels and leads to interstitial and pulmonary _____ (fibrosis, infection, edema, consolidation).

2. The type of pulmonary edema in ARDS is known as _____ (cardiogenic, noncardiogenic) pulmonary edema because it _____ (is, is not) caused by heart failure.

3. In addition to the pulmonary system, progression of ARDS involves failure of all the following organ systems **EXCEPT** the: _____ .
   A. central nervous system
   B. gastrointestinal system
   C. renal and hepatic system
   D. humoral system
   E. cardiovascular system

ETIOLOGY

4. Some common disorders leading to ARDS include all the following **EXCEPT:** _____ .
   A. shock
   B. hyperventilation
   C. trauma
   D. infection
   E. inhalation injury

5. Numerous humoral and cellular agents are responsible for the development of ARDS. Once injury has occurred in ARDS, the protein-rich fluid accumulates in the interstitium and _____ spaces about _____ (8 hours, 24 hours, 3 days) after the development of the disorder.

PATHOLOGY

6. Arrange the pathological progression of ARDS from early to late phase as follows: _____
   _____ .
   I. proliferative phase
   II. exudate phase
   III. fibrotic phase

   A. I, II, and III
   B. I, III, and II
   C. II, I, and III
   D. II, III, and I
   E. III, II, and I

7. The *exudate* phase of ARDS lasts for up to _____ (12 hours, 2 days, 7 days) and it includes all
   the following characteristics **EXCEPT:** _____ .
   A. thickening of alveolar septa
   B. endothelial cell swelling
   C. widening of intercellular junctions
   D. type 1 pneumocyte damage

8. During the *exudate* phase of ARDS, interstitial and alveolar _____ (fibrosis, edema) and
   eosinophilic hyaline membranes are developed. The lungs at this stage appear airless, edematous, heavy,
   and _____ (fibrotic, hemorrhagic).

9. Hypoxic _____ (vasodilation, vasoconstriction) develops during the *exudate*
   stage of ARDS. Along with thrombi formation and interstitial edema, the pulmonary artery pressure (PAP)
   is _____ (increased, decreased). The change in PAP during the exudate stage of ARDS is
   _____ (reversible, irreversible).

10. The *proliferative* phase of ARDS is characterized by _____ (destruction, regeneration) of the alve-
    olar epithelium.

11. The *fibrotic* phase occurs _____ (3 days, 1 week, 3 to 4 weeks) after the onset of ARDS. It is
    characterized by widespread formation of _____ (emphysema-
    tous tissues, collagenous tissues, pulmonary edema, atelectasis) causing _____
    (destruction, thickening) of the alveolar septa.

12. The *fibrotic* phase of ARDS is associated with fibrous obliteration of the pulmonary microvasculature and
    _____ (increased, decreased) arteriolar muscularization. This condition may produce prolonged
    pulmonary _____ (hypotension, hypertension).

PATHOPHYSIOLOGY

13. In ARDS, the lungs become stiff or noncompliant because interstitial and alveolar edema _____
    (increases, decreases) the surfactant concentration. In addition, damaged type II pneumocytes
    _____ (increase, decrease) the production of surfactant. As a result of these two events, microat-
    electasis develops and the lung compliance is _____ (increased, decreased) and the work of
    breathing is _____ (increased, decreased).

14. The gas exchange mechanism in ARDS is hindered due to _____ _____ (dead space ventilation, intrapulmonary shunting), a condition characterized by lack of _____ (ventilation, perfusion) in relation to the degree of _____ (ventilation, perfusion).

15. Hypoxemia caused by shunting _____ (does, does not) respond to oxygen therapy very well. This type of hypoxemia is known as _____ hypoxemia.

16. Obliteration of pulmonary microvasculature and arteriolar muscularization cause a(n) _____ (increase, decrease) of the PAP. This leads to pulmonary _____ (hypertension, hypotension) and eventual _____ (left, right) ventricular failure.

CLINICAL FEATURES

17. About 1 day after onset the initial signs of ARDS include _____ (increase, decrease) in the work of breathing, _____ (bradycardia, tachycardia), _____ (apnea, tachypnea), and cough. The chest x-ray and auscultation are _____ (normal, abnormal) at this time.

18. Because of arterial hypoxemia, the alveolar to arterial difference in oxygen tension, $P(A-a)o_2$, is _____ (increased, decreased) in the initial stage of ARDS. To compensate for this condition, the patient _____ (hyperventilates, hypoventilates) leading to uncompensated respiratory _____ (acidosis, alkalosis).

19. As ARDS progresses, intravascular fluid leaks into the interstitial and alveolar spaces causing interstitial and pulmonary _____ (fibrosis, edema), respectively. At this stage, inspiratory _____ (wheezes, crackles) are heard and the patient suffers from _____ (mild, moderate, severe) hypoxemia.

20. In severe ARDS, _____ (respiratory, metabolic, respiratory and metabolic) acidosis is often seen because of _____ (hyperventilation, hypoventilation) and _____ (aerobic, anaerobic) metabolism.

21. In stage I of ARDS, the chest radiograph shows _____ .
    A. minimal abnormalities
    B. air bronchograms
    C. interstitial emphysema
    D. interstitial and pulmonary edema

22. About 24 hours after the onset of ARDS (stage II, acute phase), the chest radiograph is characterized by _____ .
    A. air bronchograms
    B. interstitial infiltrates
    C. alveolar infiltrates
    D. A and B only
    E. all the above

23. About 1 week after the onset of ARDS (stage III, chronic phase), the alveolar fluid begins to _____ (clear, accumulate). However, interstitial edema and pulmonary interstitial emphysema may take place.

24. Pulmonary capillary wedge pressure (PCWP) is measured with a _____ (pulmonary, systemic) _____ (artery, venous) or Swan-Ganz catheter.

25. The PCWP measurement is usually _____ (normal to low, moderate to high) in ARDS patients when the cause is noncardiogenic. For patients who have cardiogenic pulmonary edema, the PCWP measurement is usually _____ (low, high).

TREATMENT

26. The treatment of ARDS is primarily supportive, to include all the following **EXCEPT:** _____
    _____ .
    A. treat precipitating problem
    B. pulmonary lavage
    C. provide adequate tissue oxygenation
    D. provide nutritional support

27. Antibiotics and vasopressors are ordered for a patient who has been diagnosed with ARDS. You would conclude that the antibiotics are used to treat _____ and vaso-pressors are prescribed to manage _____ .

28. In ARDS, tissue oxygenation _____ (can, cannot) be supported by oxygen therapy alone because of _____ (dead space ventilation, intrapulmonary shunting). Mechanical venti-lation with _____ (intermittent mandatory ventilation [IMV], pressure support ventilation [PSV], positive end-respiratory pressure [PEEP]) is usually needed.

29. Nutritional support is vital in the treatment of ARDS because malnutrition can directly affect all the follow-ing **EXCEPT**: _____ .
    A. hypoxic and hypercapnic drive
    B. muscles of ventilation
    C. immunosuppression function
    D. surfactant function
    E. neurological function

30. Mechanical ventilation with PEEP corrects _____ (dead space ventilation, shunt-ing) by reopening the atelectatic regions of the lungs. Recruitment of collapsed alveoli by this ventilation modality helps to reverse the _____ (increasing, decreasing) functional residual capacity and pulmonary compliance commonly seen in ARDS.

31. Side effects of inappropriate PEEP include barotrauma, _____ (increased, decreased) pulmonary compliance from overdistended alveoli, _____ (increased, decreased) venous return and cardiac output ($\dot{Q}T$), _____ (increased, decreased) pulmonary vascular resistance, and _____ (increased, decreased) right ventricular afterload.

32. The right ventricular afterload is the _____ (central venous pressure, pulmonary artery pressure, pulmonary capillary wedge pressure) measured by a pulmonary _____ (artery, vein) catheter.

33. Optimal (best) PEEP is one that can provide best oxygen delivery (Pa_{O_2}, O_2 saturation) at an FI_{O_2} of less than _____ (0.4, 0.6, 0.8) and with minimal _____ (increase, decrease) of cardiac output.

34. Inverse inspiratory time to expiratory time (I:E) ratio ventilation, high-frequency ventilation, and other modes of ventilation may be tried when the _____ (FI_{O_2}, PEEP, pressure sup-port, V_T, respiratory rate [RR]) with conventional ventilation fails to reverse the refractory hypoxemia in ARDS.

35. Weaning of the ventilator rate may begin when the patient's condition has stabilized, F_{IO_2} is less than _____ (0.4, 0.7, 1.0), and PEEP requirement is _____ (2, 5, 10) cm H_2O or less.

36. List the signs of weaning failure.

    _____

    _____

37. Hemodynamic status of a patient can best be monitored by a _____ (Foley, central venous, pulmonary artery) catheter. In addition to the CVP, PAP, and PCWP measurements, this catheter allows sampling of mixed venous blood and provides other fluid management functions.

38. Match the following hemodynamic measurements with the respective pressure and volume location in relation to the ventricles:

    Hemodynamic Measurements   **Pressure and Volume Ventricular Location**

    A. CVP _____   1. left ventricular preload
    B. PAP _____   2. left ventricular afterload
    C. PCWP _____   3. right ventricular preload
    D. systemic artery pressure _____   4. right ventricular afterload

    Systemic artery pressure is measured via an arterial catheter while the other three measurements are obtained via a pulmonary artery catheter.

39. Static compliance reflects the characteristics of the _____ (airways, lungs and chest wall, airways and lungs and chest wall) whereas dynamic compliance reflects the condition of the _____ (airways, lungs and chest wall, airways and lungs and chest wall).

    [**NOTES: Static** means **NO** airflow. When the airflow is absent, there is no airway resistance. Static compliance is measured during absence of airflow and it reflects the lung and chest wall compliance only. Static compliance is a form of elastic resistance (elasticity of the lungs and chest wall).

    Dynamic compliance means with airflow. When the airflow is present, airway resistance becomes a critical factor. Dynamic compliance is measured in the presence of airflow; therefore it includes airway resistance (nonelastic resistance) and lung and chest wall compliance (elastic resistance).]

    Changes in static compliance are always accompanied by similar changes in dynamic compliance. However, changes in the dynamic compliance can occur independently without corresponding changes in the static compliance. See the following questions.]

40. When the lungs and chest wall get stiffer, as in ARDS, the static compliance will _____ (increase, decrease). The dynamic compliance will _____ (increase, decrease) by about the same proportion.

41. When the airway resistance is increased, as in asthma, the static compliance will _____ _____ (increase, decrease, have little or no change) while the dynamic compliance will _____ (increase, decrease) independently.

CHAPTER **14**

CHEST TRAUMA

INTRODUCTION

1. Suicide, homicide, accidental falls, and motor vehicle accidents (MVAs) are the most common causes of _____ (chest trauma, trauma-related deaths)

2. Rank from highest (1) to lowest (4) incidence of injury that may occur as a result of chest trauma.
   A. _____ hemothorax
   B. _____ lung parenchyma
   C. _____ chest wall
   D. _____ pneumothorax

ETIOLOGY

3. Chest trauma may be caused by blunt or penetrating injuries. Classify and match the type of injury with the incidence of chest trauma injury as follows:

Type of Injury

A. blunt trauma _____
B. penetrating injury _____

Incidence

1. fall from a building
2. bullet wound
3. MVA
4. knife wound
5. metal fragments from and explosion

INJURY PATHOPHYSIOLOGY

Chest Wall Injuries

4. A common occurrence with chest wall injury is _____ (panlobular, centrilobular, subcutaneous) emphysema. This means that air is present _____ (in the pleural cavity, under the skin).

5. A chest wound that acts as a one-way valve to the movement of air or gases is called _____
   _____ .

   A. spontaneous pneumothorax
   B. tension pneumothorax
   C. subcutaneous emphysema

6. Clavicular fractures may cause clinical problems if the bony ends _____
   _____ .
   A. puncture the lung
   B. penetrate underlying blood vessels
   C. lacerate the brachial nerve plexus
   D. A and B only
   E. all the above

7. A _____ (higher, lower) incidence in rib fractures is seen in adults than in children because the
   ribs of _____ (older, younger) patients are more brittle and easier to break on forceful impact as
   seen in chest wall injuries.

8. Fracture of _____ (cervical vertebrae 1 and 2, ribs 1 and 2) in chest trauma is
   rare because they are protected by the tissue and bones of the shoulders.

9. Ribs 5 through 9 are usually fractured on forceful impact to the _____ (anterior, posterior) aspect
   and the _____ (midclavicular, midaxillary) line of the chest.

10. Localized high intensity impacts to the chest may cause penetration of the pleural space. This may result
    in any of the following conditions **EXCEPT:** _____ .
    A. pleural effusion
    B. pneumothorax
    C. hemothorax
    D. hemopneumothorax

11. Abdominal injuries resulting from fractured ribs are most often associated with fractures of ribs
    _____ (1 through 5, 5 through 9, 9 through 11).

12. Fractured ribs may cause pain, guarded cough, atelectasis, and shallow breathing. List *five* other complica-
    tions that may occur with multiple rib fractures.

    _____

    _____

    _____

    _____

    _____

13. The most common sites for sternal injuries occur along the junction of the manubrium and the sternal body
    or transversely through the sternal body. These injuries are associated with all the following conditions
    with the **EXCEPTION** of: _____ .
    A. rupture of the great vessels
    B. cardiac contusions
    C. abdominal injuries
    D. flail chest
    E. tracheobronchial rupture

14. _____ (Chest trauma, Flail chest, Pulmonary contusion) is
    defined as two or more fractures along the same rib in three or more adjacent ribs. Under this condition,
    the affected side of the chest wall _____ (expands, contracts) during inspiration and
    _____ (expands, contracts) during expiration. This is called _____
    movement of the chest wall.

15. The paradoxical movement of flail chest is more pronounced as respiratory effort is magnified due to _____ (increasing, decreasing) compliance or _____ (increasing, decreasing) $\dot{V}/\dot{Q}$ mismatch.

Lung Parenchymal Injuries

16. Match each of the following *three* terms with its respective meaning:

    A. pneumothorax _____   1. blood and air in the pleural cavity
    B. hemothorax _____   2. air in the pleural cavity
    C. hemopneumothorax _____   3. blood in the pleural cavity

17. Blunt chest trauma may lead to pneumothorax, hemothorax, or hemopneumothorax. This condition is usually caused by penetration of the lungs and tearing of intercostal arteries by the _____ _____ .

18. Blood or air in the pleural space can _____ (increase, reduce) the effective lung volumes.

19. Decreased lung volumes due to accumulation of blood and air in the pleural space can lead to _____ .

    A. decreased intrapulmonary shunt
    B. bronchopleural fistula.
    C. vesicular breath sounds
    D. increased $\dot{V}/\dot{Q}$ mismatch

20. In pneumothorax, the physiologic impairment becomes clinically significant when it causes _____ (10, 20, 30) percent or more reduction in total lung volume.

21. The hallmark sign of bronchopleural fistula is persistent _____ (air leak, fluid drainage) into the pleural space.

22. Pulmonary contusion is usually localized to the area of lung underlying the impact site of _____ (blunt, penetrating) chest trauma.

23. Intrabronchial bleeding and asphyxia is mostly likely caused by _____ (head injury, penetrating chest trauma).

24. A common event with the trauma patient is gastric aspiration. In turn, gastric aspiration may cause _____ .

    I. pneumothorax
    II. airway obstruction
    III. aspiration pneumonitis in the gravity dependent regions
    IV. pleural effusion
    V. hemopneumothorax

    A. I, III, and V only
    B. II and III only
    C. II, III, and IV only
    D. III and IV only

Airway Injuries

25. Impact injury to the larynx may produce all the following conditions **EXCEPT:** _____
    _____ .
    A. cricotracheal dislocation
    B. airway occlusion from edema
    C. vocal cord damage
    D. crushed larynx

26. The inability to lay supine is one of many symptoms of trauma to the larynx or trachea. List *five* other symptoms that may indicate laryngeal or tracheal injury.

    _____

    _____

    _____

    _____

    _____

27. Inspiratory stridor due to tracheal injury only becomes apparent when _____ (10 to 30, 30 to 50, 70 to 80) percent of the airway is occluded. The best noninvasive procedure for diagnosis of tracheal injury is _____ .
    A. direct visualization by laryngoscopy
    B. computerized tomography (CT) scan
    C. lateral neck radiograph
    D. fiberoptic bronchoscopy

Heart and Great Vessel Injuries

28. Gunshot and knife wounds to the chest cause _____ (blunt, penetrating) chest injuries.

29. Beck's triad (hypotension, muffled heart sounds, and jugular vein distension) is usually associated with _____ (myocardial contusion, cardiac tamponade, pleural effusion) when the hypotension is **NOT** caused by severe blood loss.

30. (Cardiac tamponade, Myocardial contusion) _____ may exhibit pathological changes (e.g., hemodynamic instability) similar to that caused by myocardial infarction (MI). Electrocardiograph (ECG) monitor or 12-lead ECG may be used to detect arrhythmias, ST segment _____ (elevation, depression), T-wave changes and premature ventricular contractions (PVCs).

31. In reviewing a patient's chart for a case study, you find that the patient, who expired almost immediately on entering the emergency department, was in severe shock and profound hypotension. Chest radiography of the patient shows a widened mediastinum. These signs are consistent with _____
    _____ .
    A. cardiac tamponade
    B. tension pneumothorax
    C. aortic rupture
    D. multiple myocardial contusion

Diaphragmatic Injuries

32. (Blunt, Penetrating) _____ chest trauma is the leading cause of diaphragmatic injuries. Diaphragmatic injuries may reduce lung volume by _____ (bowel, liver) herniation into the thorax. The treatment for diaphragmatic hernia is _____ .

Delayed Complications of Chest Wall Trauma

33. The most common delayed or prolonged complications of chest wall trauma is _____
_____ .

    I. septicemia
    II. atelectasis
    III. widened mediastinum
    IV. chronic pain

    A. I, II, and IV
    B. II and III
    C. II and V
    D. II, III, and V

CLINICAL FEATURES

34. You are the evening shift respiratory therapy supervisor and are called to the emergency department to assist the physician with a patient involved in an MVA. The physician asks you for a rapid assessment of a 31-year-old man with chest trauma. You would evaluate which of the following procedures? (Select *one or more* of the following choices):
    A. lung scan
    B. blood pressure
    C. symmetrical chest movement
    D. breath sounds
    E. breath efforts
    F. complete blood count
    G. Babinski reflex
    H. presence of subcutaneous emphysema

35. Revised trauma score is a scoring system that incorporates the Glasgow coma scale and it is used to evaluate the survivability of the trauma patient. A score of _____ (3, 6, 12) is associated with 99.5 percent survival among trauma patients whereas a score of _____ (3, 6, 12) is associated with only 63 percent of survival.

36. Review the revised trauma score table and continue.

Revised Trauma Score

Glasgow Coma Scale	Systolic Blood Pressure	Respiratory Rate (RR)	Points
13–15	Greater than 89 mm Hg	10–29 bpm	4
9–12	76–89 mm Hg	Greater than 29 bpm	3
6–8	50–75 mm Hg	6–9 bpm.	2
4–5	1–49 mm Hg	1–5 bpm.	1
3	0 mm Hg	0 bpm.	0

Calculate the revised trauma score for each of the following three patients:

Patient Data

Patient A	Patient B	Patient C
Glasgow score = 13	Glasgow score = 5	Glasgow score = 10
Systolic BP = 102 mm Hg	Systolic BP = 40 mm Hg	Systolic BP = 87 mm Hg
RR = 11	RR = 7	RR = 11
Trauma score = _____ .	Trauma score = _____ .	Trauma score = _____ .

37. Patient _____ (A, B, C) has the worst prognosis based on the revised trauma score.

TREATMENT

38. Acute care for chest trauma patients includes placement of central and peripheral intravenous (IV) lines, chest tubes, and a pulmonary artery catheter. Fluid balance should also be maintained. Choose other additional measures that may also be indicated for chest trauma patients.
    I. patent airway
    II. thoracotomy
    III. mechanical ventilation
    IV. lung scan
    V. hyperbaric oxygenation

    A. I, II, and III
    B. I, II, III, and V
    C. I and III
    D. III, IV, and V

39. List *three* reasons why an endotracheal tube is preferred in emergency situations.

    _____

    _____

    _____

40. You are an evening shift respiratory therapist assigned to the emergency department in a 650-bed university hospital. At 10:30 P.M. you are called by the emergency department, alerting you to an incoming trauma patient who has sustained severe facial trauma from an MVA. On initial examination, the physical signs indicate that the patient is in respiratory failure and unable to ventilate adequately. Blood gases show that immediate intubation and mechanical ventilation are indicated. Oral and nasal intubations have been attempted many times but without success.

    Which of the following would be indicated to facilitate rapid establishment of a patent airway? _____
    _____ .
    A. muscle relaxant
    B. sedative
    C. cricothyrotomy
    D. nasal continuous positive airway pressure (CPAP)

41. Ventilatory support is required for patients who are in acute or impending ventilatory (respiratory) failure. The need for mechanical ventilation is present when all the following have taken place **EXCEPT:**
    _____ .
    A. apnea
    B. Pao_2 less than 80 mm Hg
    C. $Paco_2$ greater than 50 mm Hg
    D. pH less than 7.2

42. You have been asked by the emergency department physician to intubate and place a chest trauma patient on mechanical ventilation. The patient is 32 years old and 5 ft 5 in (165 cm) tall, and weighs 154 lb (70 kg). You would proceed and select the following initial ventilator settings: _____ (Select A, B, C, or D):

Mode	Rate	Tidal Volume (Vt) (mL)	F_{IO_2}	I:E Ratio
A. Assist control	8	900	1	2:1
B. Assist control	18	700	0.5	1:1
C. Synchronized intermittent mandatory ventilation (SIMV)	20	600	0.4	1:4
D. SIMV	15	800	1	1:3

43. Positive end-expiratory pressure (PEEP) is frequently used to increase oxygenation and lung volumes. However, one of the side effects of PEEP is barotrauma and _____ (hypertension, hypotension).

44. In patients with adult respiratory distress syndrome (ARDS), the peak airway pressure required to maintain adequate oxygenation and ventilation is usually greatly _____ (increased, decreased). Which of the following ventilation techniques may be tried to reduce the peak airway pressure?
   A. CPAP
   B. inverse-ratio ventilation (IRV)
   C. pressure support IRV
   D. pressure-controlled IRV

45. Extracorporeal membrane oxygenation (ECMO) is believed to offer greater benefit to the _____ _____ .
   A. adult patients
   B. pediatric patients
   C. chronic obstructive pulmonary disease (COPD) patients
   D. A and B only
   E. all the above

Other Techniques of Respiratory Care

46. A chest trauma patient may occasionally require additional therapies. Match the following techniques with the appropriate applications:

Technique	Application
A. bronchodilator	1. hydrates secretions
B. chest physiotherapy	2. removes secretions and re-expands atelectatic lung
C. aerosol and humidity	3. reduces airway resistance

CHAPTER **15**

POSTOPERATIVE ATELECTASIS

INTRODUCTION

1. Atelectasis means _____ .
   A. air in the pleural space
   B. fluid in the pleural space
   C. hyperinflation of the lung
   D. collapsed regions of the lung

2. Mr. King is undergoing preoperative evaluation the night before his scheduled hernia operation. Which of the following risk factors would place him at the greatest risk of postoperative atelectasis? _____
   _____ .
   A. history of chronic obstructive pulmonary disease (COPD)
   B. history of cardiac disease
   C. abdominal surgery
   D. thoracic surgery
   E. use of general anesthesia

ETIOLOGY

Inadequate Lung Distension

[**NOTES:** Three factors contribute to the development of atelectasis. They are (1) inadequate lung distension, (2) obstruction of the airways, and (3) surfactant depletion.]

3. Expansion of the lungs is dependent on the ability of the respiratory muscles to generate adequate _____ (positive, negative) intrapleural pressures. A more negative intrapleural pressure generates a _____ (larger, smaller) lung volume.

4. Elderly or very sick patients develop atelectasis because they are unable to breath deep and cough, primarily due to _____ (poor coordination, lack of strength).

5. Mr. Lyons has a chronic case of kyphoscoliosis. His lungs are more prone to develop atelectasis because of the restriction or limitation placed on the movement of his _____ (thoracic cage, hemidiaphragms, accessory muscles).

6. The effectiveness of lung expansion may be compromised in patients who are obese or have neuromuscular defects. This condition limits or hinders the proper functions of the _____
   A. chest wall
   B. lungs
   C. hemidiaphragms
   D. apneustic breathing centers

7. In older and malnourished patients, their ability to generate sufficient inspiratory pressures is limited. As a result of this condition, they may not be able to _____ (deep breathe and cough, breathe at a rate greater than 12 bpm).

8. A patient asks you why he or she is unable to cough effectively. You would explain to the patient that to have an effective cough, he or she must first generate sufficient _____ (positive, negative) inspiratory force so that a large _____ (tidal volume [VT], vital capacity, functional residual capacity) may be used to force the air out rapidly.

9. Lung expansion may be compromised by kyphosis or scoliosis because this type of impairment _____ _____
   A. restricts chest wall movement
   B. affects the respiratory centers
   C. causes bronchospasm
   D. produces excessive secretions

10. When a patient undergoes surgery and receives anesthetics, the diaphragm is _____ (relaxed, tightened) and displaced _____ (upward, downward). This restrictive condition of the diaphragm _____ (limits, increases) the lung volumes and capacities.

11. In the surgical intensive care unit (SICU), there are four patients recovering from their respective operations. Which of the following surgical procedures poses the *greatest* risk of developing postoperative atelectasis? _____ .
    A. thoracic surgery
    B. upper abdominal surgery
    C. lower abdominal surgery
    D. amputation of left foot

12. Postoperative atelectasis may develop in patients recovering from coronary artery bypass surgery due to cooling of the left phrenic nerve. This condition causes _____ .
    A. loss of use of accessory muscles
    B. inadequate diaphragmatic movement
    C. congestive heart failure
    D. hypovolemic shock

Obstruction of the Airways

13. Postoperative atelectasis may be dependent on all the following conditions **EXCEPT:** _____ _____ .
    A. secretion retention
    B. inadequate cough
    C. overhydration during anesthesia
    D. impaired mucocilliary transport
    E. past medical history

14. Atelectasis distal to mucous plugs can be caused by use of anesthetic gases and high FIO_2. This is because the anesthetic or oxygen-rich alveolar gas is _____ (rapidly, gradually) absorbed into the pulmonary circulation.

Surfactant Depletion

15. All the following may cause the quantity and quality of surfactant to be reduced with the **EXCEPTION** of: _____ .
    A. pulmonary edema, contusion, or embolism
    B. anesthetic or smoke inhalation
    C. positive pressure ventilation
    D. pulmonary embolism
    E. prolonged high F_{IO_2} or low V_T ventilation

PATHOPHYSIOLOGY

16. Atelectasis reduces the _____ .
    A. functional residual capacity
    B. airway resistance
    C. lung compliance
    D. A and B only
    E. A and C only

17. When atelectasis occurs the $\dot{V}/\dot{Q}$ ratio decreases due to reduction of _____ (ventilation, perfusion).

18. Low compliance requires a _____ (higher, lower) alveolar distending pressure and work of breathing. In lung regions where the compliance is high (e.g., emphysema), _____ (underinflation, overinflation) of the lung may occur in mechanical ventilation.

CLINICAL FEATURES

19. Dyspnea and tachypnea are two common clinical signs in patients with postoperative atelectasis. Tachypnea is a compensatory maneuver to overcome the low _____ (airway resistance, lung compliance), a common clinical observation in atelectasis.

20. In the presence of yellow-green sputum, tachycardia and fever may indicate the existence of _____ _____ (heart failure, tension pneumothorax, air trapping, lung infection).

21. Chest auscultation is a valuable tool in patient assessment. Match the following breath sounds with the respective causes:

    Breath Sound

    A. absent or diminished
    B. late or inspiratory crackles
    C. vesicular (normal)

    Potential Cause

    1. abrupt opening of airways _____
    2. patent airways _____
    3. obstructed or collapsed _____

22. Observing chest movement can be a useful tool for patient assessment. The use of accessory muscles during spontaneous breathing indicates a significant _____ (increase, decrease) in the work of breathing. This is a sign that the lung compliance has _____ (increased, decreased).

23. In reviewing a patient's chest radiograph you notice that the mediastinum structure has shifted to the left. This observation is consistent with _____ .
    A. pleural effusion on both sides
    B. atelectasis on the right side
    C. atelectasis on the left side
    D. tension pneumothorax on the left side

24. In patients with postoperative atelectasis, arterial blood gases (ABGs) often reveal _____ (hypocapnia, hypoxemia). A mild respiratory _____ (acidosis, alkalosis) may occur as a compensatory mechanism for acute hypoxia.

25. Pre- and postsurgery _____ (blood gases, electrolytes, spirometry) is (are) helpful in evaluating the patient's lung volumes and pulmonary reserve. A decrease in vital capacity or inspiratory capacity is related to _____ (good, poor) pulmonary reserve.

26. Assessment of vital capacity and inspiratory capacity is also useful in _____ _____ (assessing the effectiveness, determining the type) of treatment for postoperative atelectasis.

TREATMENT

[NOTE: Treatment for atelectasis may include (1) lung inflation techniques, (2) secretion removal, and (3) mechanical ventilation.]

Lung Inflation Techniques

27. Ms. Brown, an ambulatory postoperative patient, has mild respiratory distress but normal oxygenation level. Her physician asks you to initiate a prophylactic treatment plan for the prevention of atelectasis. You would recommend _____ .
    A. incentive spirometry
    B. deep breathing and cough
    C. continuous positive airway pressure (CPAP)
    D. A and B only
    E. all the above

28. CPAP is indicated if the patient has intrapulmonary shunting and _____ (hypoventilation, refractory hypoxemia), one that responds poorly to _____ (ventilation, oxygen therapy).

29. Intermittent positive pressure breathing (IPPB) treatments would be indicated for patients who are unable to perform incentive spirometry and have a vital capacity of less than _____ (10 to 15, 15 to 20) mL/kg of ideal body weight.

Secretion Removal

30. A patient with postoperative atelectasis and retained secretions may first be treated by cough and deep breathing. If that proves ineffective, the next treatment would be _____ (bronchoscopy, chest physiotherapy).

31. Endotracheal suctioning, bronchoscopy, and bronchodilator treatments are also effective in removing _____ (lung abscess, retained secretions, pleural effusion) in postoperative atelectasis.

Mechanical Ventilation

32. Prolonged mechanical ventilation is usually unnecessary in postoperative patients because they are usually extubated soon after surgery. Patients who require prolonged mechanical ventilation may include all the following conditions **EXCEPT:** _____ .
    A. arrhythmias
    B. decreased cardiac output
    C. mediastinal bleeding
    D. cyanosis

CHAPTER **16**

INTERSTITIAL LUNG DISEASE

INTRODUCTION

1. Interstitial lung disease is a group of diseases that causes _____ (destruction, inflammation) and pulmonary fibrosis of the _____ (upper, lower) respiratory tract.

2. All of the following interstitial lung diseases have **NO** known etiology with the **EXCEPTION** of: _____ .
   A. idiopathic pulmonary fibrosis
   B. tuberculosis
   C. sarcoidosis
   D. rheumatoid arthritis

3. Interstitial lung disease may be caused by chronic exposure to airborne particles. The resulting conditions include all the following **EXCEPT:** _____ .
   A. histoplasmosis
   B. asbestosis
   C. silicosis
   D. pneumoconiosis
   E. hypersensitivity pneumonitis

4. Pulmonary fibrosis may be caused by the side effects of certain therapeutic treatments. List *three* such treatments.

   _____

   _____

   _____

5. The events leading to interstitial lung diseases typically follow five stages (A-E). Fill in the missing stages in the development of interstitial lung disease.
   A. injury
   ↓
   B. _____
   ↓
   C. disordered repair of involved tissue
   ↓
   D. _____
   ↓
   E. end-stage lung disease

ETIOLOGY

6. Interstitial lung diseases resulting from asbestos, silica (sand), or coal are examples of chronic exposure to _____ (organic, inorganic) airborne agents.

7. Hypersensitivity pneumonitis may develop on chronic exposure to certain organic dusts or organic _____ (antibodies, antigens).

8. _____ are bacteria that may cause hypersensitivity pneumonitis. They grow rapidly at temperatures between 45°C and 60°C (113°F and 140°F), temperatures that occur during vegetation decomposition.
   A. *Mycobacterium tuberculosis*
   B. *Escherichia coli*
   C. *Thermophilic actinomycetes*
   D. *Histoplasma capsulatum*

9. Some types of hypersensitivity pneumonitis are named after the causative organic materials. Write the primary organic source of infection for the following hypersensitivity pneumonitis:

Name of Hypersensitivity Pneumonitis	*Organic sources*
A. humidifier lung	_____
B. mushroom lung	_____
C. grain handlers lung	_____

10. Interstitial lung diseases induced by illicit street drugs or prescription drugs are rather rare. (True or False) _____ .

11. Interstitial lung disease may be a harmful side effect of _____ (cancer chemotherapy, cardiac drugs).

12. Interstitial lung diseases may develop because of the side effects of certain drugs or substances. Match the problems leading to interstitial lung disease with the sources of these drugs or substances.

Problems Leading to Interstitial Lung Disease	*Sources*
A. gas toxicity leading to pulmonary edema and adult respiratory distress syndrome (ARDS)	1. antibiotics
B. amiodarone	2. inert filler of illicit drugs
C. nitrofurantoin	3. oxygen therapy
D. talc	4. antiarrhythmics
E. heroin	5. cancer chemotherapy
F. cytosine arabinoside	6. narcotics

PATHOLOGY AND PATHOPHYSIOLOGY

[NOTES: In the event of lung injury and inflammation, immune cells are released to repair the damages of the lung tissues. The immune cells include neutrophils, eosinophils, lymphocytes, and macrophages.]

13. The first event leading to interstitial lung disease is lung injury leading to pulmonary _____ (inflammation, hypertension). This condition is characterized by _____ _____ .
    A. an influx of immune cells into the alveoli and alveolar walls
    B. a rapid onset of fluid accumulation in the liver and lower extremities
    C. development of cardiogenic pulmonary edema (ARDS)
    D. pulmonary hypertension leading to cor pulmonale

14. The immune reaction causes damage to the alveoli. Consequently, the _____ (type I, type II, type III) cells are destroyed and replaced by the surfactant-producing _____ (type I, type II, type III) cells.

15. At end-stage interstitial lung disease, the alveoli are replaced with fibrotic connective tissue and cystic air spaces that are lined with cuboidal or columnar epithelium. These cystic air spaces _____
_____ .
    A. produce pulmonary surfactant
    B. do not participate in gas exchange
    C. are filled with white blood cells
    D. are filled with pulmonary secretions

CLINICAL FEATURES

Medical History

16. Symptoms of lung involvement in interstitial lung disease are nonspecific and may resemble all the following **EXCEPT:** _____ .
    A. restrictive lung disease
    B. heart disease
    C. obstructive lung disease
    D. pulmonary vascular disease

17. Progressive dyspnea or nonproductive cough are usually found in the _____ (initial, intermediate, late) stage of interstitial disease.

18. Accumulation of fluid in the liver and extremities is found in the advanced stages of interstitial lung disease. This is a result of _____ .
    A. hypervolemic pulmonary edema
    B. pulmonary hypertension and left heart failure
    C. pulmonary, pedal, and hepatic edema
    D. pulmonary hypertension and right heart failure

19. The history of a patient is useful in determining the cause of interstitial lung disease. Which of the following are essential information in a patient's medical history? _____
_____ .
    I. hereditary diseases
    II. current and previous medications
    III. the patient's environment
    IV. the patient's workplace

    A. I, II, and III
    B. I, II, and IV
    C. II, III, and IV
    D. all the above

Physical Examination

20. *Early* in the course of interstitial lung disease the physical examination findings usually reveal tachypnea, inspiratory crackles, jugular vein distension, pedal edema, pulmonary hypertension, and digital clubbing. (True or False) _____ .

Laboratory Data

21. During the initial stage of interstitial lung disease arterial blood gases (ABGs) are normal. As the disease progresses the $P(A–a)O_2$ gradient _____ (increases, decreases) and hypoxemia on exertion or at rest may occur. During the terminal stages of pulmonary fibrosis, _____ (hypocapnia, hypercapnia) may occur due to hypoventilation and CO_2 retention.

22. The initial lung volumes and flows are normal with interstitial lung disease. As the disease progresses, pulmonary function testing usually shows a(n) _____ (obstructive, restrictive) lung disease process. This is characterized by _____ (increasing, decreasing) total lung capacity and residual volume.

23. In restrictive lung diseases, the forced expiratory volume in 1 second and forced vital capacity percent (FEV_1/FVC %) is usually _____ (increased, decreased, unchanged) because FEV_1 and FVC are both reduced simultaneously.

24. The lung compliance in interstitial lung disease is _____ (increased, decreased) due to formation of cystic air spaces and pulmonary fibrosis.

25. A significant _____ (increase, reduction) of lung diffusion capacity (D_{LCO}) is a(n) _____ (early, late) indicator of the presence of interstitial lung disease.

26. In patients with interstitial lung disease, desaturation of the hemoglobin during exercise is a _____ (rare, common) finding. This is primarily due to _____ _____ .

    A. increase of lung volumes
    B. decrease in shunting
    C. increase of ventilation
    D. increase in $\dot{V}/\dot{Q}$ mismatch

27. Early in the development of interstitial lung disease chest x-rays may have the following patterns: _____ .

    I. loss of vascular markings on the affected side
    II. ground glass appearance on chest radiography
    III. blunting of costophrenic angles
    IV. patterns of opaque nodules or lines

    A. I, II, and III
    B. I and IV
    C. II and IV
    D. III and IV

28. Gallium-67 is a radioactive isotope that is absorbed in areas of _____ (atelectasis, consolidation, inflammation) and it is used to _____ (show the location of inflammation, evaluate the effectiveness of therapy).

29. Which of the following is **NOT** indicated in verifying the presence of interstitial lung disease: _____ _____ .

    A. complete history and physical
    B. fiberoptic bronchoscopy
    C. transbronchial biopsy
    D. bronchoalveolar lavage

TREATMENT

30. The goal of treating interstitial lung disease is to prevent further irreversible lung damage. Prednisone, cyclophosphamide, and azathioprine are _____ (antibiotics, bronchodilators, immunosuppressives) used to control _____ (airway obstruction, inflammation, fluid retention).

31. To treat interstitial lung disease, supplemental oxygen is _____ (rarely, often) indicated.

CHAPTER **17**

NEUROMUSCULAR DISEASES

INTRODUCTION

1. Which of the following is **NOT** directly responsible for the proper functions of the respiratory pump? _____ .
   A. respiratory muscles
   B. respiratory center
   C. nerves
   D. peripheral sensors
   E. cardiovascular system

2. The respiratory center is an integral part of the _____ (cardio-vascular, central nervous, autonomic nervous) system.

3. Nerves that are responsible for ventilation send the impulses from the respiratory center to the _____ _____ (respiratory muscles, heart, lungs).

4. Changes of the carbon dioxide and oxygen levels in the blood are monitored or sensed by the central and peripheral sensors called _____ .

5. Ventilatory failure may result if _____ (any one, all four) of the four components (i.e., respiratory muscles, respiratory center, nerves, peripheral sensors) of the respiratory pump is (are) affected by neuromuscular disease.

RESPIRATORY CENTERS

6. The respiratory centers are located within the _____ and _____ in the brain stem.

7. The medullary respiratory center is responsible for maintaining a _____ _____ (constant tidal volume [VT] and frequency, rhythmic respiratory pattern) during breathing.

8. The VT and breathing frequency are regulated by the _____ .
   A. apneustic center
   B. pneumotaxic center
   C. medullary center
   D. A and B only
   E. all of the above

9. The respiratory centers receive information on ventilatory requirements from three types of sensors in the body. The information gathered produces impulses that travel down the spinal column and exit at various levels to innervate the neuromuscular junctions of the respiratory muscles. Match the types of sensors with the sensor locations. You may use any answer *more than once.*

Type of Sensor	*Sensor Location*
A. oxygen _____	1. cerebral cortex
B. hydrogen ions _____	2. carotid bodies
C. mechoreceptors (pressures) _____	3. brain stem
	4. lungs

CHEMORECEPTORS

10. The receptors that sense the level of carbon dioxide and oxygen in the fluid around them are called the _____ .

    A. mechanoreceptors
    B. J receptors
    C. chemoreceptors
    D. carotid bodies
    E. aortic bodies

11. The receptors located at the bifurcation of the common carotid arteries and the aorta are responsible for sensing the level of _____ (oxygen, carbon dioxide, hydrogen ion) in the blood.

12. The _____ (central, peripheral) chemoreceptors are located on the ventral surface of the medulla and they are sensitive to changes in the ionic concentration of the cerebral spinal fluid (CSF).

13. The ionic concentration of the CSF is regulated by all the following **EXCEPT:** _____ _____ .

    A. bicarbonate ions
    B. carbonic acid
    C. hydrogen ions
    D. carbon dioxide

14. Use the following terms to fill in the blanks:
    A. central chemoreceptors
    B. bicarbonate
    C. hydrogen
    D. carbon dioxide

    The blood-brain barrier closely regulates the movement of _____ and _____ ions. Because _____ can move freely across the blood-brain barrier, the _____ respond(s) mainly to the changes of the _____ in the blood.

NERVE TRANSMISSION

15. The *three* nerves that are of greatest importance to ventilation are the abdominal, intercostal, and phrenic nerves. Match the nerves to the points on the spinal column from which they arise.

Nerve	*Locations of Spinal Column*
A. abdominal _____	1. thoracic and lumbar spine
B. intercostal _____	2. C3–5
C. phrenic _____	3. T1–12

NEUROMUSCULAR JUNCTION

16. Define synapse.

_____

17. When the nerve ending is stimulated by a nerve impulse, it releases _____
at the synapse.

18. Acetylcholine (a neurotransmitter) causes the respiratory muscles to _____ (contract, relax) and
it is deactivated by an enzyme acetylcholinesterase.

RESPIRATORY MUSCLES

19. List _four_ inspiratory muscles.

_____

_____

_____

_____

20. List _four_ expiratory muscles.

_____

_____

_____

_____

[NOTES: Expiration is normally a passive process and it occurs when the lung tissues recoil during expiration. Expiratory muscles are only used during _active_ expiration such as during pursed-lip breathing or forced exhalation. In addition to the four expiratory muscles mentioned previously, the rectus abdominous muscles are also used in active expiration. There are two external abdominal muscles, one on each side, from the pubic bone to the ensiform cartilage and fifth, sixth, and seventh ribs. (Source: _Taber's Cyclopedic Medical Dictionary_, ed. 18. FA Davis Company, Philadelphia, 1997.)**]**

PATHOLOGY AND PATHOPHYSIOLOGY

Respiratory Centers

21. _____ primarily affects adults, particularly those with cerebral
vascular disease, insufficient respiratory drive, or defects of the central controllers.
A. sedative and narcotic drugs
B. central sleep apnea
C. primary alveolar hypoventilation

22. When there is no obvious defect of the respiratory pump or lungs, apnea caused by _____
_____ is common. In this type of apnea, the $Paco_2$ _____ (can, cannot) be
normalized by the patient.
A. sedative and narcotic drugs
B. central sleep apnea
C. primary alveolar hypoventilation

23. _____ can directly depress the respiratory centers and lead to
apnea.
A. sedative and narcotic drugs
B. central sleep apnea
C. primary alveolar hypoventilation

Nerve Interruption

24. Trauma frequently causes damage to the spinal cord. Nerves that arise from the spinal cord below the level
of injury become nonfunctional. For example, damage to the spinal cord at the C1-2 level will cause all
muscles and functions innervated at or _____ (above, below) C1-2 to become nonfunctional.

25. Match the spinal cord levels with the respective nerves and muscles that are associated with them.

Spinal Cord Level	Peripheral Nerve (Muscle)
A. cervical 1–2 (C1–2) _____	1. intercostal (intercostal)
B. cervical 3–5 (C3–5) _____	2. abdominal (abdominal wall)
C. cervical 4–8 (C4–8) _____	3. phrenic (diaphragm)
D. thoracic 1–12 (T1–12) _____	4. cervical (scalene)
E. thoracic 7–Lumbar 1 (T1–L1) _____	5. spinal accessory (sternocleidomastoid)

26. During coronary artery bypass surgery, excessive cooling of the _____ (cervical, phrenic) nerve
may cause paralysis of the diaphragm.

27. _____ (Amyotrophic lateral sclerosis [ALS], Poliomyelitis) is a viral infection that
causes destruction of the motor neurons in the anterior horn of the spinal column.

28. _____ (ALS, Poliomyelitis) is a disease of unknown etiology that causes degeneration of the motor neurons in the anterior horn of the spinal column. ALS is more commonly known as
_____ (Babe Ruth's, Lou Gehrig's, Hank Aaron's) disease.

29. _____ (Guillain-Barré syndrome, Myasthenia gravis) causes ascending paralysis
that destroys the myelin sheath around the peripheral nerves. This condition is usually preceded by a viral
infection.

Neuromuscular Junction

30. Botulism poisoning, myasthenia gravis, chemical warfare, or organophosphate insecticides are examples
that can cause interruption of nerve impulses at the neuromuscular junction. For each example, describe
the process leading to the problem at the neuromuscular junction.
A. botulism poisoning

_____

B. myasthenia gravis

_____

C. chemical warfare or organophosphate insecticides

_____

Muscle Diseases

31. Muscular dystrophy is caused by a _____ that leads to progressive muscular weakness and failure. In severe cases, it may lead to respiratory failure.
    A. congenital abnormality
    B. viral infection
    C. trauma-related abnormality

CLINICAL FEATURES

32. In patients with neuromuscular disease, wasting or paralysis of the *inspiratory* muscles may lead to complications. Describe the changes that may occur to a patient's (A) tidal volume (V_T), (B) respiratory rate (RR), and (C) perception of breathing.
    A. V_T _____
    B. RR _____
    C. perception of breathing _____

33. List *two* complications caused by wasting or paralysis of the *expiratory* muscles.

    _____

    _____

34. Sputum retention, mucus plugging, atelectasis, and pneumonia are common complications of neuromuscular disease due to weakness of the _____ (hemidiaphragms, inspiratory muscles, expiratory muscles) and ineffective coughs.

35. Arterial blood gas (ABG) samples may be normal with *mild* neuromuscular disease. If the disease is severe, hypoxemia becomes a common finding along with a(n) _____ (increased, decreased) pH and _____ (increased, decreased) carbon dioxide levels.

36. In adult patients with neuromuscular disease, the pulmonary function test usually reveals a vital capacity (VC) of less than _____
    A. 1.5 liters
    B. 2.5 liters
    C. 4 liters
    D. 15 percent of predicted VC

37. Maximum inspiratory pressure (MIP) is a useful tool in tracking the disease process that involves the inspiratory muscles. A MIP of _____ usually indicates severe neuromuscular involvement or poor inspiratory reserve.
    A. less than +20 to +30 cm H_2O
    B. less than −20 to −30 cm H_2O
    C. more than +20 to +30 cm H_2O
    D. more than −20 to −30 cm H_2O

    [NOTES: MIP is the same as negative inspiratory force (NIF).**]**

38. While you are tending to a patient in the medical intensive care unit (MICU), Dr. Brown asks you to measure the patient's MIP. Describe how you would instruct the patient to perform the MIP maneuver.

    _____

    _____

39. Ms. Klinkner, your patient with a history of myasthenia gravis, achieves a MIP of -40 cm H_2O. You would interpret her current inspiratory reserve as being _____ (good, poor).

40. You are a respiratory care practitioner (RCP) assigned to the medical floor. Ms. Warren, a patient recently admitted for viral pneumonia, claims that her legs feel weak and tingling. She also claims that she has trouble breathing and swallowing. All the complaints have been cumulative. You inspect the lab work and notice that the CSF protein level is 131 mg/100 mL. You would suspect Ms. Warren's condition may be due to _____ .
    A. myasthenia gravis
    B. ALS
    C. poliomyelitis
    D. Guillain-Barré syndrome
    E. botulism poisoning

41. You are the evening shift supervisor of a respiratory care department in a 250-bed hospital. You are paged by the therapist assigned to the surgery floor. The therapist informs you that the condition of one of the patients has changed since her surgery the previous day. The patient claims that she cannot read the goal markings on the incentive spirometer. She was able to see the markings in the morning but now has blurred vision and drooping eyelids. In addition, she has trouble swallowing. You relate the findings to the physician. Later the physician transfers her to ICU and orders a Tensilon test along with Q2h VC and V_T. You would conclude that the physician is trying to rule out _____

    _____ .
    A. myasthenia gravis
    B. ALS
    C. poliomyelitis
    D. Guillain-Barré syndrome
    E. botulism poisoning

42. Fasciculations and initial weakness of the distal muscle groups (e.g., hands) are two distinctive signs of _____ . The disease progresses over a period of 2 to 7 years affecting all extremities as well as the respiratory muscles. The prognosis is poor with respiratory failure as the final outcome.
    A. myasthenia gravis
    B. ALS
    C. poliomyelitis
    D. Guillain-Barré syndrome
    E. botulism poisoning

    [NOTES: The location of an injury to the spinal column will determine the extent of the respiratory involvement. Use the following table and *study* the location of spinal injury with the respective respiratory involvement.]

Location of Spinal Injury	*Respiratory Involvement*
Above C3	Near complete respiratory muscle paralysis
Between C3 and 8	Some use of respiratory muscles
Below C8	Weak expiratory muscles, ineffective cough

43. Injury to the spinal column at the _____ (C3, C6, T1, L2) level is most likely to cause acute ventilatory failure and severe hypoxia in a spontaneously breathing patient.

44. Spinal injury at a level _____ (between C3 and C8, below C8, above C3) will produce *nearly complete respiratory muscle paralysis.* The diaphragm is elevated and immobile and this condition leads to a rapid onset of respiratory acidosis and hypoxemia. The breath sounds are diminished and may be absent. A bedside vital capacity may reach up to _____ (20, 50, 70) percent of the predicted value.

45. Spinal injury at a level _____ (between C3 and C8, below C8, above C3) will cause the patient to be quadriplegic but with *some use of the respiratory muscles.* The vital capacity is diminished and it may _____ (improve, worsen) over the first 12 months following injury. Dyspnea on exertion may occur.

46. Spinal injury at a level _____ (between C3 and C8, below C8, above C3) often *affects the expiratory muscles* leading to ineffective cough and risk of secretion retention. _____ _____ (Pneumothorax, Atelectasis, Ventilatory failure, Respiratory acidosis) is a common presentation in this type of spinal injury.

47. Mr. Thomas, a patient who was thrown from a moving motor cycle without wearing a helmet, has a diagnosis of spinal injury at the C2 level. Which of the following respiratory care modalities is most likely required for this patient? _____ .
    A. nasal continuous positive airway pressure (CPAP)
    B. oxygen therapy
    C. intermittent positive pressure breathing (IPPB) therapy
    D. long-term mechanical ventilation

TREATMENT

48. Patients with neuromuscular disease usually have weakened respiratory muscles, difficulty in clearing secretions, and atelectasis. IPPB may be helpful in preventing or reversing atelectasis. List *three* other bronchial hygiene techniques that may enhance secretion removal.

    _____

    _____

    _____

49. Patients with neuromuscular disease may require intubation and mechanical ventilation when progressive dyspnea and retained secretions are present along with the following clinical measurements:
    A. vital capacity less than _____ (15, 20, 30) mL/kg
    B. respiratory rate greater than _____ (15, 20, 30) breaths per minute
    C. _____ (increasing, decreasing) Pa_{CO_2}

50. You are an RCP assigned to the ICU. Dr. Lipper asks you to perform weaning parameters on Mr. Kaolin, a patient with Guillain-Barré syndrome. He is orally intubated and has been on an intermittent mandatory ventilation (IMV) mode at a rate of 12 for almost 2 weeks. While his condition is stable, he fails to meet any of the weaning parameters. You would ask the physician to consider _____

    _____ .
    A. pressure support ventilation
    B. tracheostomy
    C. nasal CPAP
    D. inverse ratio pressure release ventilation

51. Patients with neuromuscular disease are at risk of pulmonary embolism and pneumonia. Antibiotics should be used if fever is present and intravenous _____ should be used to reduce the incidence of pulmonary embolism.

52. Weaning from mechanical ventilation can be successful when the patient is free of infection, and has stable hemodynamic status and improving respiratory muscle strength. Signs of adequate lung functions include the following measurements _____ .
    A. vital capacity greater than _____ liters
    B. maximum inspiratory pressure greater than _____ cm H_2O
    C. spontaneous V_T greater than _____ mL

53. ALS and high cervical fracture are two neuromuscular conditions that improvement of lung functions during the convalescent period is _____ (certain, unlikely).

54. Guillain-Barré syndrome is treated primarily with _____ (antibiotics, corticosteriods, supportive measures).

55. A patient with Guillain-Barré syndrome normally has very good prognosis if no serious complications develop. However close monitoring of the patient is mandatory because _____
_____ .
    A. period of stability is present in only 25 percent of all cases
    B. threat of respiratory failure is life threatening
    C. anticholinesterase drugs may cause ventilatory failure
    D. corticosteriods may cause an anaphylactic reaction and induce acute pulmonary edema

56. Patients with myasthenia gravis should be admitted to the hospital when _____
_____ (paralysis of the legs, difficulty in swallowing or breathing) occurs. The medications for myasthenia gravis include _____ (neostigmine, endrophoniumn), which is a(n) _____ (cholinergic, cholinesterase, anticholinesterase) drug.

57. There is no specific treatment for ALS other than supportive measures. Respiratory failure may occur without warning and close monitoring is indicated. If this chronic condition worsens, intermittent ventilatory support may be delivered by _____ .
    A. IPPB machines
    B. positive-pressure volume limited ventilator
    C. negative-pressure ventilator (body respirator)
    D. nasal CPAP

58. Describe the major advantage of a negative-pressure ventilator for ventilatory support of ALS.

    _____

59. The location of spinal injury will determine the extent of the patient support needed. If the injury is above _____ (C3, T1, L3), tracheostomy and long-term ventilatory support will be needed. If the injury is below _____ (C3, C5, C7), the patient may only require assistance with secretion removal and nocturnal ventilatory support.

CHAPTER **18**

BACTERIAL PNEUMONIA

INTRODUCTION

1. Pneumonia is an inflammation of the _____ (main-stem bronchi, lung parenchy-ma). It may be caused by _____ .
   A. bacterial infection
   B. viral infection
   C. fungal infection
   D. A and B only
   E. all the above

2. (Bacterial, Viral) _____ pneumonia is a common medical problem despite the availability of antibiotics.

3. Pneumonia contracted in the hospital environment is the leading cause of _____ in the hospital.
   A. ventilator dependence
   B. nosocomial deaths
   C. medical malpractice suits
   D. medical disability

ETIOLOGY

4. Sterility of the distal airways may be compromised by neuromuscular disease and acute viral upper respi-ratory infections. List *three* other factors that may compromise the sterility of the distal airways.

   _____

   _____

   _____

5. Ms. Kitchen, a patient with an admitting diagnosis of myasthenia gravis, is being evaluated for a treatment plan. The primary concern in the care of Ms. Kitchen would be her ability to _____ .
   A. cough effectively
   B. prevent aspiration
   C. breathe deep
   D. A and B
   E. all the above

6. Systemic disorders such as AIDS, cirrhosis, renal failure, malnutrition, and cancer may contribute to the development of _____ .
    A. pneumonia
    B. pleural effusion
    C. pulmonary hypertension
    D. congestive heart failure

7. Pneumonia caused by _____ is closely associated with AIDS.

8. Pathogens that cause pneumonia may enter the lungs by all the following systems **EXCEPT** the: _____ .
    A. digestive system
    B. exocrine system
    C. circulatory system
    D. pulmonary system

9. Which of the following patient conditions is *least* inducive for deposition of microbes into the lower airways? _____ .
    A. sleep apnea
    B. orally intubated
    C. recent tracheotomy
    D. diminished gag reflex

PATHOLOGY AND PATHOPHYSIOLOGY

10. Infections of the lungs can lead to inflammatory response. In turn, this response causes exudates and white blood cells to fill the _____ .
    I. interstitial space
    II. hilum area
    III. pleural space
    IV. alveolar space

    A. I and III
    B. I and IV
    C. II and III
    D. II and IV

11. Permanent damage to the lung tissues may occur if the pneumonia is caused by organisms such as *Staphylococcus* and *Pseudomonas*. This type of infection is known as a _____ (primary, secondary, necrotizing) infection.

12. The sputum culture of Mr. Kalton confirms the preliminary diagnosis of pneumonia. Due to the process of acute inflammation and consolidation of the lungs, you would anticipate all the following changes in his clinical condition **EXCEPT** a(n) _____ .
    A. increase of $\dot{V}/\dot{Q}$ mismatch
    B. decrease of ventilation
    C. decrease of shunting
    D. decrease of gas exchange

13. In providing respiratory care to Mr. Kalton during the acute stage of pneumonia, lung consolidation may exhibit all the following signs or measurements with the **EXCEPTION** of: _____ .
    A. decrease in lung compliance
    B. increase in work of breathing
    C. increase in lung volumes
    D. increase in dyspnea

CLINICAL FEATURES

Medical History

14. Mr. Lowe is a patient on the medical floor with a diagnosis of bacterial pneumonia. In evaluating his clinical condition, you would expect to find all the following signs **EXCEPT:** _____ .
    A. fever
    B. bradycardia
    C. productive cough
    D. dyspnea
    E. pleuritic chest pain

Physical Examination

15. Ms. Jones is diagnosed with bacteria pneumonia. She has numerous productive coughs that yield copious amounts of purulent sputum. Other typical findings in her physical examination may include _____ _____ (tachycardia, bradycardia) and _____ (tachypnea, apnea). These findings can be attributed to hypoxemia, _____ (high, low) compliance, or _____ (increased, decreased) metabolic rate.

16. Cyanosis is a(n) _____ (common, uncommon) occurrence in patients with pneumonia. They also have reduced chest expansion and excessive use of accessory muscles. The primary reason for these findings is due to _____ .
    A. increased compliance
    B. decreased compliance
    C. decreased airway resistance
    D. oxygen toxicity
    E. ventilatory failure

17. Match the clinical conditions related to pneumonia with the respective breath sounds. You may use any answer *more than once.*

    Clinical Conditions

    A. lung consolidation _____
    B. airway obstruction _____
    C. excessive mucus _____

    Breath Sounds

    1. inspiratory crackles
    2. coarse crackles
    3. diminished or absent
    4. bronchial breath sounds

18. One of the complications of pneumonia is pleural inflammation. This may cause a condition known as _____ (pleural friction rub, pleural effusion, emphysema).

Laboratory Data

19. The number of white blood cells in a blood sample may indicate the severity or progression of bacterial infection. The number of white blood cells is usually increased in bacterial infection and this condition is called _____ (leukocytosis, leukopenia). If the number of bands or immature white blood cells is increased, it may be indicative of a(n) _____ (abating, worsening) infection. On the other extreme, _____ (leukocytosis, leukopenia) may occur if the immune system is overwhelmed by the infection.

20. Match the clinical conditions related to pneumonia with the respective radiographic signs.

Clinical Conditions	*Radiographic Signs*
A. lung consolidation _____	1. blunting of costophrenic angle
B. pleural effusion _____	2. interstitial infiltrates
C. normal airways with lung infiltrates _____	3. bronchogram

21. Ms. Jamison, a 35-year-old patient with pneumonia, has the following arterial blood gas (ABG) results: pH 7.50, $Paco_2$ = 32 mm Hg, Pao_2 = 60 mm Hg, and Hco_3 = 22 mEq/L. This is interpreted as _____ (respiratory, metabolic) _____ (acidosis, alkalosis). This is a compensatory response to _____ .

22. In reviewing a patient's chart you notice that the physician has ordered a sputum culture and sensitivity (C & S) test. You may want to check if any antibiotic has been started for the patient. This is because a sputum sample should be collected _____ (before, after) the initiation of antibiotics. Explain why:

_____

23. Describe the clinical use of Gram's stain.

_____

24. The _____ (Gram's stain, culture and sensitivity) method of sputum analysis is used to identify the pathogen so that the most effective antibiotic may be chosen for treating the infection.

TREATMENT

25. In severe pneumonia, the patient should be admitted to the hospital. List *four supportive* measures that should be provided for the patient.

_____

_____

_____

_____

[NOTE: In treating pneumonia, diagnostic tests such as chest radiograph, sputum Gram's stain, and C & S should be done to formulate a treatment plan. Antibiotic therapy should begin as soon as possible by using Gram's stain to identify the type (Gram positive or Gram negative) of microbes involved. The more time-consuming C & S analysis of sputum should be done if a specific antibiotic is indicated for certain microbes.**]**

26. Match the antibiotics with the appropriate organisms based on Gram's stain outcome. You may use an answer *more than once.*

    Antibiotics

    A. cephalosporins _____
    B. penicillin _____
    C. ampicillin _____

    Results of Gram's Stain

    1. gram-negative coccobacilli
    2. gram-positive diplococci

27. Many nosocomial infections are Gram-_____ (negative, positive) and they are relatively resistant to antibiotics and transfer easily by contact. Proper and frequent _____ (hand, bronchial, nasal) washing is the proven method to reduce nosocomial infection.

28. During surgical or invasive procedures, _____ (aseptic, sterile, isolation) technique should always be followed to minimize the incidence of pneumonia in the hospital.

CHAPTER **19**

PNEUMONIA IN THE IMMUNOCOMPROMISED PATIENT

INTRODUCTION

1. If a person's immune system is damaged or compromised, infectious organisms that are typically _____ _____ (difficult, easy) to control and eradicate by a normal immune system may cause serious pulmonary infections.

2. Define opportunistic infections.

   _____

   _____

ETIOLOGY

Basic Function of the Immune System

3. List the *three* principle characteristics of the immune system.

   _____

   _____

   _____

4. In diseases such as rheumatoid arthritis, systemic lupus erythematosus, or scleroderma the immune system attacks the _____ (microbes, host) and these diseases are called _____ diseases.

5. The immune response detects molecules with specific shapes unique to the organism it is attacking and these uniquely shaped molecules are called _____ (antibodies, leukocytes, antigens, macrophages).

6. The immune system remembers when it has been invaded by an organism and provides a more rapid, larger response when it is invaded by the same organism a second time. This principle is called _____ memory.

Immune Cell Type	*Subdivision*	*Notes*
Lymphocytes (Congregate in spleen, thymus, and lymph nodes)	B lymphocytes (can develop into antibody secreting cells; these antibodies thus produced are called immunoglobulins [Ig]—types IgG, IgM, IgE, IgA, and IgD)	IgG replaces IgM and becomes the primary antibody to fight infection IgM is the first antibody against infection IgE mediates allergic reactions IgA inhibits binding of microbes to the mucosa
	T lymphocytes (3 kinds) (1) Natural killer cells (2) Helper T lymphocytes (3) Suppressor T cells	(1) Natural killer cells have a direct cytotoxic effect on target cells (2) Helper T lymphocytes promote the development of antibodies by B lymphocytes and assist development of natural killer cells (3) Suppressor T cells inhibit the immune responses; this effect is important to inhibit attacks on the host and to regulate immune response following antigen exposure
Monocytes (Mononuclear phagocytic white blood cells)	Monocytes are derived from the myeloid stem cells; they are short lived and have a half-life of about 1 day; they circulate in the bloodstream and move into the tissue, at which point they mature into long-lived macrophages	Lymphocytes (above) and monocytes make up the majority of immune cells
Granulocytes (polymorphonuclear leukocytes) (They are formed in the bone marrow and circulate in the blood as neutrophils, eosinophils, and basophils)	Neutrophils (the most common granulocyte; they are responsible for detecting invading microbes, phagocytosing, killing, and degrading them) Eosinophils (these granulocytes make up 1% to 3% of the white blood count; their activity is not entirely clear but they are known to destroy parasitic organisms and to play a major role in allergic reactions; they release some chemical mediators that cause bronchoconstriction) Basophils (these granulocytes make up less than 1% of the white blood count; they are essential to the nonspecific immune response to inflammation)	Low number of circulating neutrophils in blood (less than 500/µL) indicates immunosuppression)

Anatomy of the Immune System

7. Immune cells are _____ (confined to a few organs of, scattered throughout) the body and they are mobilized and circulated to specific areas as they are needed.

8. Name the *three* major types of immune cells.

   _____

   _____

   _____

9. Lymphocytes and monocytes make up the majority of the immune cells. (True or False) _____ .

10. List *three* locations where the majority of lymphocytes are found.

   _____

   _____

   _____

11. _____ (B lymphocytes, T lymphocytes) can develop into antibody-secreting cells and these antibodies thus produced are called _____ .

12. Name the *five* types of immunoglobulins (Ig).

   _____

13. The primary function of _____ (IgA, IgE, IgD, IgG, IgM) is to act as the first antibody against infection.

14. The primary function of _____ (IgA, IgE, IgD, IgG) is to replace IgM and become the primary antibody to fight infection

15. The primary function of _____ (IgA, IgE, IgD, IgG, IgM) is to mediate allergic reactions.

16. The primary function of _____ (IgA, IgE, IgD, IgG, IgM) is to inhibit binding of microbes to the mucosa, thus forming an initial barrier to entry of microorganisms across the mucosa.

17. Name the *three* types of T lymphocytes.

   _____

   _____

   _____

18. The primary function of the _____ (natural killer cells, helper T lymphocytes, suppressor T cells) is to inhibit the immune responses and attacks on the host, and to regulate immune response following antigen exposure.

19. The primary function of the _____ (natural killer cells, helper T lymphocytes, suppressor T cells) is to produce a direct cytotoxic effect on target cells.

20. The primary function of the _____ (helper T lymphocytes, suppressor T cells) is to promote the development of antibodies by B lymphocytes and assist the development of natural killer cells.

21. Helper T lymphocytes are a significant factor in _____ (autoim-munity, cell-mediated immunity) that is responsible for defense against specific types of organisms (e.g., *Mycobacterium tuberculosis*).

22. The mononuclear phagocytic white blood cells are known as _____ _____ (leukocytes, lymphocytes, monocytes, eosinophils).

23. Monocytes are derived from the myeloid stem cells and they are _____ (long lived, short lived). They circulate in the bloodstream and move into the _____ at which point they mature into _____ (long-lived, short-lived) macrophages.

24. Granulocytes are also called _____ leukocytes.

25. Name *three* major polymorphonuclear cells.

_____

_____

_____

26. Granulocytes are formed in the _____ and circulate in the blood as neutrophils, eosinophils, and basophils.

27. _____ (Basophils, Eosinophils, Neutrophils) are the most common granulocyte.

28. What are the primary functions of neutrophils?

_____

29. Because _____ (basophils, eosinophils, neutrophils) are the most common granulocyte, the low number of these granulocytes in blood (less than _____/µL) is indicative of immunosuppression.

30. _____ (Basophils, Eosinophils, Neutrophils) make up 1 to 3 percent of the white blood count. They are known to destroy parasitic organisms and to play a major role in allergic reactions. They release some chemical mediators that cause _____ (bronchodilation, bron-choconstriction).

31. _____ (Basophils, Eosinophils, Neutrophils) are granulocytes that make up less than 1 percent of the white blood count. They are essential to the nonspecific immune response to inflam-mation.

PATHOLOGY AND PATHOPHYSIOLOGY

32. When a patient's immune system is depressed or malfunctioning, the patient is _____ (more, less) likely to develop infections.

33. Antibody deficiency is a cause of immunodepression and development of disease. This is because an inad-equate level of antibodies _____ (increases, decreases) a patient's susceptibility to infections.

34. In patients with an antibody deficiency, infections are _____ (more, less) frequent and _____ (more, less) severe than they would be if the immune system were normal.

35. Infections in patients with antibody deficiency _____ (are, are not) typically classified as opportunistic because they may occur in patients with normal immunity.

36. Name two common bacteria that may lead to repeated infections in patients with a complete or partial absence of antibodies.

_____

_____

37. According to the textbook, the most *severe* form of antibody deficiency is _____ _____ (X-linked agammaglobulinemia, selective IgA deficiency) and the most *common* form is _____ (X-linked agammaglobulinemia, selective IgA deficiency).

38. Defects in cellular immunity are another cause of immunodepression and development of disease. Name a common disease that is caused by a defect of cell-mediated immunity.

_____

39. Defects in phagocyte function are another cause of immunodepression and development of disease. This condition becomes evident when the circulating _____ (eosinophils, neutrophils, basophils) are _____ (more than, less than) 500/dL.

40. Define neutropenia.

_____

_____

41. Acquired neutropenia is frequently caused by _____ .

CLINICAL FEATURES

42. On physical examination, opportunistic pneumonias have signs and symptoms that are _____ _____ (different from, similar to) other common pneumonias.

43. List the common symptoms of opportunistic pneumonia.

_____

_____

44. Describe the additional signs and symptoms of pyogenic pneumonia.

_____

_____

_____

_____

45. Immunosuppression may be documented by the following laboratory results: an abnormally _____ (high, low) number of lymphocytes, particularly CD4+ cells; _____ (neutrocytosis, neutropenia); _____ (increase, decrease) in the A–a gradient or $P(A–a)_{O_2}$; and _____ (increase, decrease) in lung density on chest radiographs.

46. List *four* types of microbes that may infect an immunocompromised patient.

_____

_____

_____

_____

47. Culture and microscopic examination of the sputum are the _____ (most, least) invasive and _____ (most, least) readily available technique to identify an infectious agent.

48. Gram stain is used to identify the _____ of the microbes and acid fast stain is done to identify_____ .

49. A stain should also be performed for *Pneumocystis carinii* if the patient has a defect in his _____ , as seen in deficiency of T lymphocytes.

50. Describe the suggested procedure to collect a sputum specimen.

_____

_____

51. List *three* options for obtaining a "better" sputum specimen if the saline-induced specimen cannot identify the organism.

_____

_____

_____

52. Name the microbe that causes the acquired immunodeficiency syndrome (AIDS).

_____

53. The human immunodeficiency virus (HIV) preferentially infects cells that have the _____ antigen; and as the infection progresses, the helper T lymphocytes that express this antigen are destroyed.

54. The immune system becomes compromised when the numbers of helper T cells decrease from a normal concentration of _____ to _____/mL to below _____/mL.

55. List *three* microbes that cause common opportunistic pulmonary infections in patients with AIDS.

_____

_____

_____

56. List *four* nonopportunistic pulmonary infections in patients with AIDS.

_____

_____

_____

_____

57. List *two* forms of cancer in patients with AIDS.

_____

_____

58. List at least *five* symptoms of patients with AIDS.

_____

_____

_____

_____

_____

59. Examination of the respiratory tract of AIDS patients may reveal _____ (black, white, purple) plaques on the tongue and in the mouth. This oral thrush is due to infection of the mucocutaneous tissue by a _____ (bacteria, virus, fungus) called _____ .

60. Define transplant rejection.

_____

_____

61. Cyclosporin is a medicine used to control transplant rejection by _____ (enhancing, suppressing) a patient's immune system. Therefore, this type of medicine _____ (increases, decreases) the likelihood of pulmonary infection.

62. List *three* signs of post-transplantation infection.

_____

_____

_____

63. Neutropenia means an abnormally _____ (high, low) level of neutrophils in blood.

64. Because cells that generate hair and white blood cells are very _____ (sensitive, insensitive) to chemotherapy, chemotherapy _____ (often, seldomly) causes hair loss and neutropenia.

65. Neutropenia is evident when the granulocyte count is less than _____/mL and this condition usually occurs _____ (1, 7, 14, 30) days after initiating chemotherapy and continues for 2 to 3 weeks.

66. During the period of neutropenia a patient is prone to develop infections. Explain why.

_____

_____

67. Fever is a very important sign of infection in a neutropenic patient because this is often the initial clue of a serious _____ (organ failure, ventilatory failure, infection, sepsis).

68. Drugs such as corticosteriods, cyclophosphamide, or azothioprim decrease the risk for both opportunistic and nonopportunistic pneumonia. (True or False) _____.

TREATMENT

69. Define empirical treatment.

_____

70. Empirical drug therapy is selected based on the specific immune defect of the patient. In general, a patient with neutropenia is usually treated with _____ against pyogenic bacteria such as *P. aerugenosa* or fungi such as *Aspergillus* organisms.

71. Patients with AIDS are usually empirically treated with the combination of _____ and _____ because they are likely to have Pneumocystis pneumonia.

72. Describe the specific drug therapy to treat infections caused by *P. carinii.*

_____

_____

_____

_____

_____

_____

73. For most immunocompromised patients with a fungal pneumonia, _____ is the first line of drugs. Oral antifungal agents classified as _____ are also effective for this type of fungal infection.

74. Drugs such as itraconazole, ketoconazole, and fluconazole are reserved for use against _____ (mild, severe) infections or for patients who have responded well to amphotericin B, but further oral therapy is desired.

75. Patients who develop tuberculosis and have AIDS require intensive therapy with multiple drugs. Name the *four* drugs that should be used during the first 2 months of drug therapy.

_____

_____

_____

_____

76. Name the *two* drugs that should be used to treat patients with tuberculosis and AIDS during the remaining 7 months after the initial 2 months of drug therapy.

_____

77. Explain the reason for providing prophylactic drug therapy to patients with immunodeficiencies such as AIDS.

_____

_____

78. Antibiotics should be started to prevent *Pneumocystis* pneumonia when the number of CD4+ lymphocytes is _____ (more, less) than _____/mL.

79. The first choice for prophylactic treatment is a daily tablet of _____ and _____. If the patient cannot tolerate this tablet, aerosolized _____ or _____ tablets may be used.

80. Rifampin and clarithromycin are recommended for prevention of *M. avium* complex if the CD4+ count is below _____ (100, 200, 300, 400)/mL.

CHAPTER **20**

TUBERCULOSIS

INTRODUCTION

1. Pulmonary tuberculosis has been eradicated since the 1950s. (True or False) _____ .

2. Which of the following statements about tuberculosis (TB) is **NOT** true? _____
   _____ .
   A. TB kills more people than all other infectious diseases combined.
   B. TB causes more than 30 percent of AIDS-related deaths.
   C. TB infects one new person every minute.
   D. One third of the world's population is infected with TB.

3. The incidence of TB in the United States is affected by all the following factors **EXCEPT:** _____
   _____ .
   A. population demographics
   B. inadequate health-care access
   C. ineffective antimicrobial drugs
   D. malnutrition
   E. institutional housing

ETIOLOGY AND TRANSMISSION

4. The microbe that causes TB is called _____ .

5. Describe the general characteristics of *Mycobacterium tuberculosis*.

   _____

   _____

   _____

6. Because *M. tuberculosis* is a(n) _____ (aerobe, anaerobe), it grows best in areas of the body
   where the partial pressure of oxygen is the _____ (highest, lowest). Therefore, cavitation of the
   lung is usually seen in the _____ (upper, lower) lobes.

7. *M. tuberculosis* is transmitted by _____ .
   A. aerosolized droplets
   B. body fluid contact
   C. sexual transmission
   D. blood transfusion
   E. contaminated medical supplies

8. Define fomites.

_____

PATHOLOGY AND PATHOGENESIS

9. Inhaled mycobacteria settles in the distal parenchyma of the lung and slowly migrates by way of the
_____ and _____
systems throughout the body.

10. About _____ (1 to 2, 3 to 4, 6 to 8) weeks after the initial infection the host's immune system
causes localized inflammation, and containment of the infection by formation of _____ .

11. A granuloma develops in the infected lung tissue and results in a fibrin mass with necrosis and parenchymal breakdown forming a cheesy material at the center known as _____ .

12. The initial lung lesion is called a _____ nodule and the combination of the initial lung lesion and the affected lymph node is known as the _____ .

13. The initial stage of TB is _____ (easy, difficult) to detect on a chest radiograph because the
lesions may be seen as _____ (large, small), sharply defined opacities.

14. The initial stage of TB usually _____ (heals completely, worsens) in the majority of infected individuals _____ (leaving small, leading to large) scars, which
may calcify later.

15. The body's cell-mediated immune response is usually _____ (effective, ineffective) in controlling
the mycobacterial infection in the initial stage. _____ (Essentially, Not) all the bacteria will have
been killed.

16. Some surviving bacilli may lay dormant in either the primary or the metastatic sites, sometimes for many
years, until some event results in reactivation and reinfection. (True or False) _____.

17. Between the primary and reinfection phases is a dormant or healthy period known as
_____ .
   A. active TB
   B. TB infection without disease
   C. passive TB

18. Between the primary and reinfection phases, there is _____ (clear, no) evidence of disease and
a _____ (positive, negative) skin test is seen.

19. A positive reaction to the TB skin test indicates the presence of _____ (live, dead) tuberculin
bacilli in the body.

20. List at least *three* predisposing factors that may lead to postprimary (reactivation) infection.

_____

_____

_____

21. During the period of postprimary or reactivation infection, fibrosis and cavity formation takes place leading to a(n) _____ (increase, decrease) of lung volume.

22. Retractions and change in lung volume _____ (usually, seldomly) affect the shape and integrity of the large airways.

23. Describe the changes of the bronchi due to retractions of the lungs in pulmonary TB.

    _____

    _____

24. Define miliary TB.

    _____

    _____

25. In spite of the continuous destruction of infected lung parenchyma and loss of lung volume, the ventilation and perfusion *ratio* is not severely affected. Explain why.

    _____

    _____

    _____

26. In pulmonary TB, hypoxemia and hypercapnia are _____ (common, unusual) _____ (when, unless) the patient has concurrent lung disease such as chronic obstructive airways disease.

27. As the TB progresses, pulmonary function testing would reveal a(n) _____ (increase, decrease) of lung volumes and flow rates.

28. To rule out TB, the patient interview should include several key questions. List at least *three*.

    _____

    _____

    _____

29. List at least *six* common complaints of a patient with TB.

    _____

    _____

    _____

    _____

    _____

    _____

30. Physical examination findings in the patient with TB _____ (are, are not) specific enough to make the diagnosis. For this reason, a physical examination is done to determine the _____ (presence, extent) of the disease.

31. Together with bacteriologic examinations of sputum and a positive skin test, the chest radiograph provides a valuable tool in the diagnosis of tuberculosis. (True or False) _____ .

32. Because many non-TB strains of mycobacteria can show up on _____ (Gram stain, acid-fast smears), a culture of _____ is necessary for confirmation of TB.

33. The use of xylocaine during bronchoscopy can alter the outcome of a sputum sample. Explain.

_____

_____

34. The Mantoux skin test for TB is an _____ (intramuscular, intravenous, intracutaneous) injection of a standardized dose of purified protein derivative (PPD).

35. A _____ (positive, negative) reaction to the PPD relies on a visible or palpable induration (raised, hardened area) caused by prior sensitization of the TB organism.

36. According to the CDC classification of positive skin test reactions, induration of 10 mm or greater is the standard of a positive test result for all patients. (True or False) _____.

37. Induration of 5 mm or more is considered a positive PPD skin test for certain patient populations. List *one*.

_____

38. Induration of 10 mm or more is considered a positive PPD skin test for certain patient populations. List at least *three*.

_____

_____

_____

39. Induration of 15 mm or more is considered a positive PPD skin test for certain patient populations. List *one*.

_____

40. PPD skin testing for TB infection is recommended in high-risk populations. List at least *three* groups of individuals for whom skin testing is recommended.

_____

_____

_____

41. The absence of an induration or reaction to the tuberculin test _____ (does, does not) exclude the diagnosis of TB or TB infection.

TREATMENT

42. The first line of drugs for TB is considered effective and relatively low risk for toxic side effects. Name the drugs and treatment criteria for TB in a 6-month regimen.

_____

_____

43. Name the drugs and treatment criteria for TB in a 9-month regimen.

_____

_____

44. Regimens of _____ (more than 9 months, less than 6 months) are not recommended for treatment of TB.

45. The most common side effect of rifampin, isonicotinic acid hydrazide (INH), and pyrazinamide is _____ and this condition can be avoided by stopping treatment when _____ (cardiac, pancreatic, liver) enzymes reach three to five times upper limits of normal.

46. _____ (Isoniazid, Pyrazinamide, Rifampin) has the potential side effects of gastrointestinal (GI) upset, skin eruptions, flu-like symptoms, and red-orange discoloration of urine and other body fluids.

47. Directly observed chemotherapy is done to ensure appropriate treatment by _____ _____ (recording, dispensing, watching) that their TB patients _____ (take, receive) each dose of the medications.

48. The risk benefit ratio of prophylactic therapy mandates _____ (3, 6, 9) months of drug therapy for any patient with a positive TB skin test _____ (over, under) 35 years of age and for patients _____ (over, under) 35 who have a *recent* TB skin test conversion.

CHAPTER **21**

LUNG CANCER

INTRODUCTION

1. With over 30 years of medical advances in the diagnosis and treatment of lung cancer, the survival rate has shown _____ (significant increase, little change).

2. Differentiate between primary and metastatic malignancy.

   _____

   _____

ETIOLOGY

3. The association of bronchogenic cancer and cigarette smoking _____ (has, has not) been very well established. The risk and development of cancer is related to the _____
   _____ .
   I. age when smoking started
   II. number of cigarettes smoked
   III. years smoked
   IV. depth of inhalation
   V. tar and nicotine content

   A. I, II, III, and V
   B. II, and III
   C. II, III, and IV
   D. III, IV, and V
   E. all of the above

4. Prolonged exposure to passive or secondhand smoke causes a _____ (twofold, no significant) increase in the risk and development of lung cancer.

5. Asbestos, chromium, nickel, uranium, vinyl chloride, bismochloromethyl ether, and decay products of radon gas have been associated with an increase in the incidence of lung cancer. Many of these agents also _____ .
   A. cause allergic reaction
   B. potentiate the carcinogenic effects of smoking
   C. lead to congestive heart failure
   D. induce pneumonia

PATHOLOGY

6. Lung cancers are usually classified as either _____ or
_____ . The nonsmall cell carcinomas include *three* of the following **EXCEPT:** _____ .
   A. bronchocarcinomas
   B. squamous cell carcinomas
   C. adenocarcinomas
   D. large cell carcinomas

7. _____ is a type of lung cancer that often arises from the bronchial lining and it may grow and obstruct the airways.
   A. large cell carcinomas
   B. small cell carcinomas
   C. squamous cell carcinomas
   D. adenocarcinomas

8. _____ may be a primary or metastatic lung cancer. In the metastatic form, it is spread to the lungs from other organs in the body.
   A. large cell carcinomas
   B. small cell carcinomas
   C. squamous cell carcinomas
   D. adenocarcinomas

9. _____ are responsible for 15 percent of all lung cancer. They are described as having an abundant cytoplasm and may exhibit a gland-like structure and produce some mucin (a glycoprotein found in mucus).
   A. large cell carcinomas
   B. small cell carcinomas
   C. squamous cell carcinomas
   D. adenocarcinomas

10. _____ contain little cytoplasms and they grow rapidly and metastasize to distant tissues (e.g., brain and liver).
   A. large cell carcinomas
   B. small cell carcinomas
   C. squamous cell carcinomas
   D. adenocarcinomas

11. In patients with lung cancer, their pulmonary function is dependent on the size and location of lung tumors. Small peripheral tumors may have no effect on lung function but large tumors may cause all the following problems **EXCEPT:** _____ .
   A. airway obstruction
   B. retained secretions
   C. hypocapnia
   D. decreased gas exchange
   E. reduced lung volume

CLINICAL FEATURES

12. Mr. Jackson, a patient who has been diagnosed with lung cancer, is admitted to the surgical floor for prelobectomy evaluation and care. List *six* major clinical features that you would expect to find during the evaluation.

_____

_____

_____

_____

_____

_____

13. A 46-year-old, 80-pack-year smoker complains of dyspnea and chest pain. She also reports productive cough with bloody sputum. These may be the _____ (initial, terminal) signs of lung cancer.

14. Other signs that may be indicative of lung tumor development include all the following **EXCEPT** change in the: _____ .
    A. previously effective therapy
    B. quality or quantity of sputum
    C. quality of a cough
    D. electrocardiogram tracings

15. Patient complaint of shortness of breath is common when the airway or ventilation mechanism is hindered by lung tumor. Match each of the following conditions with the respective cause of dyspnea.

Condition	_Cause of Dyspnea_
A. tumor obstructs or compresses a large airway _____	1. loss of diaphragmatic function
B. tumor compresses phrenic nerve _____	2. loss of effective lung volume
C. pleural effusion _____	3. airflow obstruction

16. In reviewing the medical history of a patient who has been diagnosed with lung cancer, you note that the patient had many episodes of hemoptysis. This condition is most likely caused by _____ _____ .
    A. ulceration of the digestive tract
    B. inflammation of the sinus
    C. rupture of the capillaries of the bronchial mucosa
    D. chronic use of Bronkosol

17. Chest pain in lung cancer may be due to local involvement of any of the following areas **EXCEPT** the _____ .
    A. pleura
    B. hilar region
    C. ribs
    D. nerves

18. Partial obstruction of an otherwise normal airway may cause _____ (stridor, wheezes, crackles).

19. If breath sounds reveal wheezing that is monophonic, is localized, and does not disappear after a good cough, you may suspect the possibility of _____ .
    A. chronic bronchitis
    B. partial airway obstruction
    C. bilateral pneumonia
    D. empyema

20. In performing diagnostic chest percussion, it reveals decreased resonance over the effected areas. This may occur in all the following cases **EXCEPT:** _____ .
    A. tension pneumothorax
    B. pleural effusions
    C. lung tumors
    D. pneumonia

METASTATIC DISEASE

21. A metastatic disease is one that originates in _____

    _____ .
    A. the lungs
    B. an organ and is spread by the respiratory system or body fluids
    C. an organ and is transferred by the lymphatic or circulatory system to another organ

Nonspecific Systemic Symptoms

22. Anorexia, weight loss, nausea, vomiting, and weakness are some _____ (specific, nonspecific) indicators of lung cancer. These symptoms generally provide a very _____ (good, poor) prognostic sign.

Intrathoracic Spread

23. Tumor spread within the chest follows many different pathways. Match the following types of spread with the appropriate process:

Type of Spread	Process
A. brachial neuritis _____	1. phrenic nerve involvement
B. unilateral hemidiaphragmatic paralysis _____	2. obstruction of lymph flow resulting in fluid accumulation between visceral and parietal pleura
C. superior vena cava syndrome _____	
D. pleural effusion _____	3. extension of tumor into the pericardium and epicardium
E. pressure on the recurrent laryngeal nerve _____	4. disruption of the laryngeal nerve by tumor or enlarged lymph nodes
F. pericardial effusion _____	5. growth of tumor through the parietal pleura and into the brachial plexus
	6. compression or direct invasion of the great veins in the thoracic outlet

Extrathoracic Spread

24. Lung cancer may involve extrathoracic sites including the skin and lymphatics. List *six* other common sites of extrathoracic spread of tumor.

    _____

    _____

    _____

    _____

    _____

    _____

DIAGNOSIS

25. Along with the presence of risk factors, there are at least *three* official *screening* processes for lung cancer. (True or False) _____ .

Radiographic Data

26. To be visible on the chest radiograph a tumor must be at least _____ (2 to 3 cm, 2 to 3 mm) in size.

27. Lung tumors that are large enough for biopsy sampling via the fluoroscopic transthoracic needle aspiration method should be at least _____ (1 to 2 cm, 1 to 2 mm) in size.

28. Because malignant lung tumors grow rapidly, precise measurement of their diameters on chest radiograph is extremely important because a tumor doubles in volume with an increase of the diameter by a factor of

    _____.

    A. 1.27
    B. 2
    C. 4.04
    D. 10

    The following table shows a small increase in the diameter of a sphere (from 1 to 1.27 cm) can double its volume (from 0.52 to 1.07 cm³):

Diameter of Tumor (cm)	Radius (cm)	Volume of Tumor (cm³)
1	0.5	$4\pi(0.5)^3/3 = 0.52$
1.27	0.635	$4\pi(0.635)^3/3 = 1.07$

29. Name the method or procedure used in determining the type of lung tumor.

    _____

Laboratory Studies

Review the following table and associate the laboratory findings with the respective implications:

Possible Implications	Laboratory Findings
A. ectopic antidiuretic hormone	1. hyponatremia
B. metastatic tumor spread to bone	2. hypercalcemia
C. metastatic tumor spread to bone	3. alkaline phosphatase
D. tumor spread to liver	4. liver dysfunction
E. tumor spread to bone marrow	5. anemia, thrombocytopenia, pancytopenia
F. pericardial effusion or conduction block	6. electrocardiogram (ECG, low voltage or pulsus alternans)
G. endocarditis	7. heart murmur
H. tumor spread to lymphatic system	8. restrictive lung disease
I. $\dot{V}/\dot{Q}$ mismatch or intrapulmonary shunting	9. hypoxemia

30. Define and explain the purpose of a cytology sample.

    _____

    _____

Diagnostic Procedures

31. Sputum cytology is useful in the diagnosis of _____·_____ (central squamous cell, small cell) carcinomas and it is _____ (also, not) useful in the diagnosis of peripheral lesions or solitary nodules.

32. List *six* problems associated with collecting, analyzing, or interpreting sputum cytology samples.

    _____

    _____

    _____

    _____

    _____

    _____

33. Because the sputum sample comes from the airways, cytology study is _____ (most suitable, not suited) for peripheral lesions or solitary nodules of the lungs.

34. Define and explain the use of fiberoptic bronchoscope.

    _____

    _____

35. **Transbronchial forceps** under fluoroscopic guidance can perform forceps biopsy, bronchial brushings, and washings. This diagnostic method is more successful in diagnosing _____ (bronchogenic, peripheral and parenchymal) lesions. **Fiberoptic bronchoscopy** can perform the same procedures and is better suited for diagnosing _____ (bronchogenic, peripheral) lesions.

    [**NOTES**: Study and differentiate the following techniques in obtaining a sample for diagnosis of lung cancer.]

Transbronchial forceps biopsies	Collection of tissue samples in the airway with a small forceps
Transbronchial brushings	Collection of tissue samples in the airway by use of a brush
Transbronchial washings	Collection of tissue samples in the airway by washing and suctioning
Transbronchial needle aspiration biopsy (TNAB)	Collection of tissue samples in the lungs by use of a needle attached to a syringe

36. Percutaneous transthoracic needle aspiration biopsy (TNAB) is useful in the diagnosis of _____ (central, peripheral) pulmonary nodules and tumors _____ (proximal, distal) from the mediastinum.

37. A positive pleural _____ (pressure, fluid cytology, blood sample) is indicative of the spread of cancer to the pleural space.

STAGING

38. By international convention, the TNM classification system for lung cancer has been adopted by physicians world wide. This system is used to _____ .
A. classify the type of lesions
B. select appropriate therapy
C. classify the structure of lesions
D. estimate the size of the lesion

39. Define T, N, and M of the TNM tumor staging system.

T _____

N _____

M _____

40. By using the TNM classification system match the following stages with the appropriate therapy:

Stages

A. stages I and II _____
B. stage IIIA _____
C. stages IIIb and IV _____

Therapy

1. high risk surgery
2. not resectable, may be treated with radiation, with or without chemotherapy
3. resectable

TREATMENT AND PROGNOSIS

41. All of the following may be used as indexes of long-term survival for patients with lung cancer with the **EXCEPTION** of the: _____ .
A. TNM classification system
B. Karnofsky performance scale
C. Eastern Cooperative Oncology Group (ECOG)
D. Zubrod performance scale

Surgery

42. Surgical resection is the treatment of choice for patients with _____ (nonsmall cell, small cell) lung cancer that is classified as _____ .
A. stage I
B. stage II
C. stage IIIA
D. A and B only
E. all the above

43. Radiation therapy is usually selected to treat stage _____ (I, II, IIIA, IIIB), especially if the patient presents with pain, hemoptysis, or airway obstruction.

44. Chemotherapy combined with radiation therapy _____ (has, has not) substantially improved survival rates. When chemotherapy is used alone, it generally provides brief partial _____ _____ .

Radiation Therapy

45. Radiation therapy is considered a(n) _____ (effective cure, primary treatment) for patients with operable and inoperable nonsmall cell lung cancer (NSCLC).

Chemotherapy

46. Chemotherapy _____ (is, is not) recommended for small cell lung cancer. For nonsmall cell lung cancer, chemotherapy may be used as additional therapy after surgery.

Preoperative Evaluation

47. Postoperative survival of lung cancer depends on an adequate preoperative _____ _____ (nutritional status, pulmonary reserve, exercise tolerance). The desired preoperative forced expiratory volume in one second (FEV_1) should be greater than _____ .

[**NOTE:** Postoperative FEV_1 = Preoperative $FEV_1 \times (1 - \%$ resection)]

48. Mr. Jones, a patient with lung cancer undergoing lobectomy, has a preoperative FEV_1 of 2.0 liters. After a 40 percent lung resection, the estimated postoperative FEV_1 at full recovery should be about _____ liter(s) .
    A. 0.8
    B. 1.0
    C. 1.2
    D. 2.0

CHAPTER **22**

SLEEP APNEA

Clinical Definitions of Sleep Apnea

Lack of breathing during sleep that
1. lasts at least 10 seconds per episode, *and*
2. occurs more than 30 times in 7 hours of sleep

Interpretation	*Sleep Index*
1. mild sleep apnea	5 to 20 apnea episodes per hour of sleep
2. moderate sleep apnea	21 to 40 apnea episodes per hour of sleep
3. severe sleep apnea	more than 40 apnea episodes per hour of sleep

1. During a 7-hour period, the polysomnogram done on a patient in a sleep laboratory shows 20 apnea episodes that lasted more than 10 seconds each time. This finding _____ (is, is not) consistent with the clinical diagnosis of sleep apnea. Based on the criteria of sleep index, this finding is _____ (insignificant, significant) because the sleep index is based on the number of apnea episodes per hour of sleep.

2. In reviewing a patient's polysomnogram, you notice that the highest number of apnea episodes in a 1-hour period is seven. You would classify this as _____ (mild, moderate, severe) sleep apnea.

3. Mr. Wells, a patient who has recently been diagnosed with sleep apnea, asks you to explain the meaning of his diagnosis. You would tell him that this clinical diagnosis is based on the cessation of breathing that lasts at least _____ seconds each time and occurs more than _____ times in _____ hours of sleep.

4. Name the *three* types of sleep apnea.

   _____

   _____

   _____

5. _____ (Obstructive, Central, Mixed) sleep apnea is evident when a patient's respiratory drive is intact but the upper airway becomes obstructed intermittently.

6. _____ (Obstructive, Central, Mixed) sleep apnea is the proper term to use when a patient's respiratory drive is absent intermittently while the upper airway is normal and patent.

7. Mixed apnea is a combination of _____ and _____ apnea.

8. A breathing pattern in which the tidal volume (V_T) and respiratory rate are not sufficient to meet the metabolic needs of the body is called _____ (hyperventilation, apnea, hypopnea).

9. Respiratory disturbance index is the _____ (sum, difference) of the number of sleep apnea episodes and _____ per hour of sleep.

10. During a traditional sleep study, all the following patient parameters are monitored with the **EXCEPTION** of: _____.
    A. eye and leg movements
    B. pulse oximetry
    C. electroencephalogram (EEG) and electrocardiogram (ECG)
    D. respiratory pattern
    E. arterial and mixed venous blood gases

11. Polysomnogram is a printout or paper record made by a _____ (single-channel, multichannel) recorder.

12. The multiple sleep latency test (MSLT) is used to assess _____ (daytime, night-time) somnolence.

13. Sleep latency is done during the patient's normal _____ (sleeping, waking) hours and it measures the amount of time from when the patient reclines in bed to when sleep occurs. If the patient takes less than _____ (5, 20, 60) minutes to fall asleep during the sleep latency test, excessive daytime sleepiness is present and it is abnormal .

SLEEP AND BREATHING

14. Name the *two* types of normal sleep.

    _____

    _____

15. Match the stages of sleep with the respective characteristics of sleep.

    Stage of Sleep

    A. stage 1 nonrapid eye movement (NREM) _____
    B. stage 2 NREM _____
    C. stages 3 and 4 NREM delta or slow-wave _____
    D. rapid eye movement (REM) stage
    _____

    Characteristic

    1. deepest level of sleep, difficult to arouse (lasts about 90 minutes)
    2. lightest level of sleep, easy to arouse (lasts 5 to 7 minutes)
    3. active sleep, increase cerebral and autonomic activities, dreaming occurs that lasts 10 to 20 minutes
    4. sleep spindles and K complexes on EEG tracings

16. Match the stages of sleep with the respective breathing patterns.

    Stages of Sleep

    A. stages 1 and 2 NREM
    B. stages 3 and 4 NREM delta or slow-wave
    C. REM stage

    Breathing Pattern

    1. irregular breathing pattern due to chemical and mechanical stimuli; short apneas of 15 seconds or less is common
    2. regular breathing pattern with 1 to 2 L decrease in minute ventilation
    3. irregular breathing pattern (similar to Cheyne-Stokes) due to loss of normal stimulatory effects and decreased metabolic rate

17. During NREM and REM sleep, there is a general _____ (increase, decrease) of skeletal muscle tone throughout the body. This condition explains the _____ (increase, decrease) in ventilation during certain stages of sleep.

ETIOLOGY

18. Ms. Faulkner, a patient who has been diagnosed with obstructive sleep apnea, is being evaluated for a treatment plan. Which of the following factors would **NOT** be contributory to her diagnosis? _____ _____ .
    A. chronic lung disease
    B. large tongue
    C. small lower jaw
    D. obesity
    E. enlarged tonsils

19. Obstructive sleep apnea occurs when the muscles of the upper airway are _____ (tightened, relaxed) during _____ (light, deep) sleep. This requires a larger negative inspiratory pressure to overcome the obstruction and leads to persistent occlusion of the upper airway.

PATHOPHYSIOLOGY

20. Apnea causes the Pa_{O_2} to _____ (fall, rise) and the Pa_{CO_2} to _____ (fall, rise). Ventilatory drive _____ (stops, returns) at this point because of the sudden changes of Pa_{O_2} and Pa_{CO_2} and stimulation of the central and peripheral chemoreceptors. These changes arouse the patient from a _____ (deeper, lighter) stage of sleep to a _____ (deeper, lighter) stage.

21. After ventilation is resumed and the patient goes back to a _____ (deeper, lighter) stage of sleep, sleep apnea occurs again.

22. This sequence of alternating apnea (deep sleep) and ventilation (arousal and light sleep) can occur hundreds of times each night. As a result of these frequent interruptions, sleep is very fragmented and the patient _____ (does, does not) feel rested in the morning.

23. At the onset of apnea and hypoxemia, bradycardia usually occurs due to _____ (vagal, sympathetic) stimulation.

24. Once breathing resumes, _____ (arrhythmia, persistent bradycardia, tachycardia) is the typical response because of diminished vagal stimulation and increased sympathetic activities.

25. _____ (Systemic, Pulmonary, Systemic and pulmonary) hypertension is a common observation in patients with obstructive sleep apnea (OSA). Therefore, the patient usually has _____ _____ (normal, higher than normal, lower than normal) systemic blood pressure and _____ (normal, higher than normal, lower than normal) pulmonary artery pressure (PAP).

26. Cardiac arrhythmias during sleep are extremely rare in OSA patients. (True or False) _____ .

CLINICAL FEATURES

Medical History

27. Patients with obstructive sleep apnea (OSA) usually have a medical history of _____ (daytime, nighttime) sleepiness and fatigue. This is primarily caused by _____ (inadequate, excessive) sleep during normal sleep hours.

28. Due to the anatomic structure of the upper airway, some patients may obtain relief from OSA by sleeping in a _____ (prone, supine, lateral) position.

29. A patient is being evaluated for the presence and severity of obstructive sleep apnea in the sleep laboratory. The patient's medical history may reveal all the following findings with the **EXCEPTION** of: _____ .
    A. productive coughs
    B. poor memory and loss of concentration
    C. headache on waking
    D. loud snoring
    E. falling asleep while driving

Physical Examination

30. Physical examination of patients with obstructive sleep apnea may reveal *one or more* of the following findings **EXCEPT:** _____ .
    A. skinny built
    B. short neck
    C. enlarged tonsils
    D. large tongue
    E. small lower jaw

31. In chronic cases of severe sleep apnea, jugular vein distension, hepatomegaly, and loud P_2 heart sound may be found. These are signs of _____.
    A. chronic lung disease
    B. cor pulmonale
    C. obesity
    D. malnutrition
    E. alcoholism

32. Hypoxemia and hypercapnia are two common findings in patients with sleep apnea because of chronic alveolar _____ (hyperventilation, hypoventilation). Arterial blood gases (ABGs) would show compensated or partially compensated _____ (respiratory, metabolic) _____ (acidosis, alkalosis).

Clinical Polysomnography

33. Polysomnogram may be used to _____ of sleep apnea.
    A. diagnose the presence
    B. evaluate the effectiveness of treatment
    C. assess the severity
    D. A and B only
    E. all of the above

34. Match the equipment used in polysomnography with the respective events monitored in sleep apnea.

Equipment

A. surface electromyography (intercostal muscle and diaphragm) _____
B. pulse oximetry _____
C. ECG _____
D. EEG _____
E. electrooculogram _____

Event Monitored

1. bradycardia and rebound tachycardia
2. delta waves and sleep stages
3. oxygen saturation
4. onset of REM sleep
5. respiratory pattern

TREATMENT

35. Treatment of patients with obstructive sleep apnea (OSA) depends on the degree of hypoxemia and severity of clinical symptoms. Match the severity of OSA with the respective clinical symptoms.

Severity of OSA

A. mild _____
B. moderate _____
C. severe _____

Clinical Symptom

1. persistent daytime sleepiness; falling asleep in routine daily functions
2. minimal daytime sleepiness
3. sleepiness during life-endangering events; signs of heart failure

36. Match the severity of OSA with the respective treatments. Use only *two of four* answers provided.

Severity of OSA

A. mild _____
B. moderate to severe _____

OSA Treatments

1. trial of continuous positive airway pressure (CPAP)
   avoidance of alcohol
   weight reduction
2. no treatment needed
3. weight reduction
   avoidance of alcohol
   sleep in lateral position
4. mechanical ventilation with pressure support

CHAPTER **23**

CROUP AND EPIGLOTTITIS

INTRODUCTION

1. Croup and epiglottitis are two conditions that generally affect children and cause _____ _____ (widening, narrowing) of the upper airway and _____ (increased, decreased) work of breathing.

2. Croup is a _____ (viral, bacterial) infection of the area _____ (below, above) the glottis. It usually affects infants and children between 6 months and _____ (1, 3, 5, 12) years of age.

3. Epiglottitis is a _____ (viral, bacterial) infection of the area _____ (below, above) the glottis; therefore it is also called supraglottitis. It affects children between the ages of (1 and 5, 3 and 8, 1 and 10) years, and occasionally infants and adults.

CROUP

Etiology

4. The most common microbes that cause croup are almost always _____ (bacteria, viruses, fungi). They may be any of the following **EXCEPT:** _____.
   A. adenovirus
   B. respiratory syncytial virus
   C. parainfluenza viruses 1 and 3
   D. *Haemophilus influenzae*
   E. influenza viruses A and B

Pathology and Pathophysiology

5. Croup causes inflammation and swelling of the anatomical structures _____ (above, below) the glottis including the larynx, trachea, and _____ (esophagus, pharynx, bronchi). Because these three areas are commonly affected, croup is also known as _____ _____ .

6. In croup, ventilation-perfusion ($\dot{V}/\dot{Q}$) mismatch and hypoxemia may occur as a direct result of _____ (dead space ventilation, airway obstruction, intrapulmonary shunting).

7. When severe airway obstruction occurs in croup, patients often experience a(n) _____ (increased, decreased) level of work of breathing. Arterial blood gases (ABGs) would show a(n) _____ (increased, decreased) $Paco_2$ and a(n) _____ (increased, decreased) Pao_2.

Clinical Features

8. The onset of croup is _____ (fast, slow) and it is usually preceded by _____ _____ (less than 12 hours, 1 to 2 days, 1 week) of fever, nasal congestion, and coughing.

9. The onset of croup is characterized by severe coughs that carry a bold or barking quality. Hoarseness is also common in croup and this condition indicates inflammation of the _____ _____ .
   A. vocal cords
   B. pharynx
   C. larynx
   D. A and B only
   E. A and C only

10. Other clinical features of croup may include all the following with the **EXCEPTION** of: _____ _____ .
    A. retraction
    B. inspiratory and expiratory stridor
    C. tachypnea
    D. diminished sensorium
    E. bradycardia

Treatment

11. Match the respiratory care treatments for croup with the respective clinical goals of these treatments.

Treatments	*Clinical Goals*
A. cool mist and oxygen _____ B. racemic epinephrine _____ C. corticosteroids _____	1. treats swelling of subglottic structures by its anti-inflammatory action 2. improves ventilation and oxygenation 3. provides temporary relief from airway edema by its vasoconstrictive action

12. Antibiotics are generally _____ (effective, ineffective) in the treatment of croup because it is a _____ (bacterial, viral) infection.

EPIGLOTTITIS

Etiology

13. Epiglottitis is a _____ (seasonal, year-round) _____ (bacterial, viral) infection commonly caused by type B *H. influenzae* and occasionally *Staphylococcus aureus*.

    [**NOTES:** *H. influenzae* are small, rod-shaped, Gram-negative bacilli; and *S. aureus* are clusters of round, Gram-positive cocci.]

Pathology and Pathophysiology

14. Epiglottitis is the inflammation of the epiglottis, aryepiglottic folds, and arytenoids (Figure 23-1 of textbook). Under direct visual examination, the epiglottis has a bright _____ (cherry red, brownish red, pinkish white) color.

15. Patients with epiglottitis often complain of difficulty in _____ (hearing, swallowing, talking) due to inflammation and swelling of the supraglottic structures.

16. Without proper and timely interventions, severe _____ (atelectasis, airway obstruction, pneumonia) can develop in epiglottitis that can lead to immediate asphyxia and ventilatory failure.

Clinical Features

17. Epiglottitis usually has a _____ (sudden, gradual) onset and patients may complain of fever, sore throat, and difficulty swallowing.

18. Direct visual examination of the epiglottis should be done when equipment and personnel are readily available to perform _____ (tracheostomy, intubation, defribillation). This is because the potential risk of complete _____ (airway obstruction, heart block) during epiglottis examination.

19. Epiglottitis is characterized by a(n) _____ (elevated, reduced) white blood count. The presence of epiglottitis can be confirmed with a(n) _____ (anterior-posterior [A-P], posterior-anterior [P-A], lateral) _____ (chest, neck) radiograph.

Treatment

20. Performing intubation or tracheostomy on patients with epiglottitis should be done under a(n) _____ (elective, controlled) environment because of the severity and rapid progression of complete airway obstruction.

21. Culture specimens from the epiglottis should be obtained _____ (before, after) placement of an artificial airway. Culture is done to determine and select the proper _____ (bronchodilator, antibiotic, mucolytic) for the treatment of epiglottitis.

[NOTES: Culture and sensitivity are usually requested together when culture of the epiglottis is indicated. Sensitivity refers to the reaction of microbes to antimicrobial drugs.]

22. The initial antibiotics for acute epiglottitis include intravenous _____ 200 to 400 mg/kg per day and _____ 100 mg/kg per day in divided doses every 4 to 6 hours for 7 to 10 days.

[NOTES: Epiglottitis may be treated by ampicillin alone unless the organism is resistant to ampicillin (β-lactamase resistant), in which case use chloramphenicol. If the organism is not susceptible to either of these drugs, use cefotaxime or ceftriaxone. *H. influenzae* vaccine may be used to prevent *H. influenzae* type b infection when child is 2 years of age or older. (Source: *Taber's Cyclopedic Medical Dictionary*, ed. 18. F. A. Davis Publishers, Philadelphia, 1997, with permission.)]

23. Extubation is the normal course of event for epiglottitis after 24 to 48 hours of treatment. The clinical signs of improvement include subsided fever and _____ (leak, no leak) around the endotracheal or tracheostomy tube.

24. For patients recovering from epiglottitis, a leaky endotracheal or tracheostomy tube can be a(n) _____ (good, bad) sign because this means that the inflammation and swelling of the epiglottis has _____ (improved, worsened).

CHAPTER **24**

RESPIRATORY SYNCYTIAL VIRUS

1. Respiratory syncytial virus (RSV) is a(n)_____ (common, uncommon) viral pathogen in infancy and early childhood.

2. RSV is the leading cause of _____ in infants and young children.
    A. pneumonia
    B. bronchiolitis
    C. epiglottitis
    D. A and B only
    E. all of the above

3. The RSV causes cells to _____ (break up, fuse together) to form a multinucleated mass of protoplasm (syncytium), thus its name *syncytial* virus.

4. The age group that is most prone to be infected by RSV is between _____ (1 to 4 weeks, 4 weeks to 1 year, 1 to 3 years) of age.

5. Newborns during the first 4 weeks after birth are less likely to be infected by RSV because of protection from _____ (maternal, infant) antibodies.

6. The common mode(s) of transmission of RSV is (are) direct contact with contaminated _____ _____ .
    A. aerosol particles
    B. secretions
    C. food and drink
    D. A and B only
    E. all of the above

7. After acquiring the RSV, the incubation period for the virus is from _____ (1 to 2, 2 to 8, 8 to 14) days.

8. RSV _____ (is, is not) very contagious because the virus remains _____ (infective, dormant) on common materials in the patient's room (e.g., clothing, paper products).

9. RSV can stay infective in nasal secretions for more than _____ (30 minutes, 6 hours, 24 hours).

PATHOLOGY AND PATHOPHYSIOLOGY

10. Complete the blanks in the following flowchart that outlines the *pathology* of RSV:

> A. RSV spread along the respiratory tract via _____ transfer

↓

> B. Peribronchiolar mononuclear infiltration and _____ of the small airway epithelium

↓

> C. _____ of bronchiole walls, submucosa, and adventitial tissue

↓

> D. Sloughing of necrotic tissues into the _____, edema, and accumulation of _____

↓

> E. _____ (Decrease) in the diameter of the airway

11. Complete the blanks in the following flowchart that outlines the *pathophysiology* of RSV:

> A. _____ of the narrowed airway by mucus

↓

> B. _____ and atelectasis in different regions of the lungs

↓

> C. _____ on exhalation due to airway obstruction

↓

> D. $\dot{V}/\dot{Q}$ mismatch, hypoxemia, _____ lung compliance, _____ airway resistance and work of breathing

CLINICAL FEATURES

12. The clinical features of RSV vary with the age of the patient and the severity of the illness. Some risk factors that increase the severity of RSV include all the following **EXCEPT:** _____ .

    A. congenital heart disease
    B. bronchopulmonary dysplasia (BPD)
    C. prematurity
    D. immunodeficient or immunosuppression
    E. metabolic acidosis

History of Present Illness

13. In RSV, the patient history often reveals contact or exposure to others who have cold symptoms or confirmed RSV infection. Before the onset of RSV, these patients often have symptoms of upper respiratory tract infection to include all the following **EXCEPT:** _____ .
    A. mild runny nose
    B. pharyngitis
    C. high fever
    D. cough

Physical Examination

14. On physical examination, patients who are infected with RSV often show the following signs with the **EXCEPTION** of: _____ .
    A. bradycardia
    B. increased work of breathing
    C. tachypnea
    D. appearance of shortness of breath

15. An infant who has a diagnosis of RSV infection shows intercostal retractions, nasal flaring, and grunting while breathing spontaneously. These are three cardinal signs of increased _____ _____ (lung compliance, work of breathing, oxygenation, airway conductance).

    [NOTES: Intercostal retractions, nasal flaring, and grunting are also the clinical signs of respiratory distress syndrome (RDS). However, the primary cause of RDS is prematurity and surfactant deficiency.**]**

16. Apneic episodes are sometimes observed during RSV infection. This is probably due to immaturity of the central respiratory control mechanism. Therefore, apneic events are more likely to be seen in infants who _____ (are premature, have congenital heart disease, are born in a breeched position).

17. Because of the retained secretions and narrowed airways in patients with RSV infection, the typical breath sounds may include all the following **EXCEPT:** _____ .
    A. crackles
    B. vesicular
    C. wheezes
    D. diminished

18. Match the following types of breath sound with the respective causes:

Breath Sounds	Potential Causes
A. wheezes _____	1. decreased gas flow due to hyperinflation of the lungs
B. diminished _____	2. retained secretions
C. stridor _____	3. narrowed trachea or larynx
D. fine crackles (during late inspiration) _____	4. narrowed airways due to inflammation and edema
E. coarse crackles (during inspiration and expiration) _____	5. obstructed airways due to atelectasis

Laboratory Data

19. For each of the following blood counts, write *normal, increase,* or *decrease* to the respective changes observed in RSV infection.

Blood Count	Change During RSV Infection
A. complete blood count _____	1. _____
B. white blood cell count _____	2. _____
C. immature white blood cell count _____	3. _____

   [NOTES: Immature white blood cells are also called **blasts** (e.g., lymphoblasts, myeloblasts). The number of blasts is increased during an infection because these cells are released in large quantity.]

20. In RSV infection, the oxygenation levels (Pa_{O_2}, O_2 content, O_2 saturation) are usually _____ (normal, increased, decreased).

21. In the acute stage of RSV infection, the patient's initial ventilatory level is _____ (normal, increased, decreased) when the respiratory muscles try to compensate for hypoxia by _____ (hyperventilation, hypoventilation). This compensatory mechanism causes the Pa_{CO_2} to be _____ (increased, decreased).

22. Jenny Camp, a 6-month-old infant diagnosed with RSV, has been in the pediatric unit for 5 days. Her arterial blood gases (ABGs) over the past 3 days are shown in the following table. You may conclude that her increasing Pa_{CO_2} is due to fatigue of the respiratory _____ (centers, muscles) and eventual _____ (hyperventilation, hypoventilation).

	pH	Pa_{CO_2}	Pa_{O_2}	F_{IO_2}
Day 3	7.38	42	58	0.3
Day 4	7.36	46	55	0.4
Day 5	7.33	52	40	0.5

23. The chest radiograph of Jenny Camp shows hyperinflation of the lungs. This becomes evident when the hemidiaphragms are _____ (elevated, flattened). Furthermore, you would expect to see _____ (widened, narrowed) intercostal spaces, and _____ (increased, decreased) anteroposterior (AP) diameter.

24. Areas of increased density on a chest radiograph typically indicate _____ (subcutaneous emphysema, tension pneumothorax, interstitial pneumonitis).

Diagnosis

25. The positive diagnosis of RSV infection is by isolation of the virus or its antigen from the _____ _____ (blood, urine, respiratory secretions). The sample may be obtained by _____ _____ (syringe and needle, Foley catheter, nasal washing or swab).

26. Once the specimen is obtained, detection of the virus should be done _____ _____ (within 12 hours, as soon as possible) by one of the immunofluorescent techniques such as enzyme-linked immunosorbent assay (ELISA).

TREATMENT

27. Match the treatments for RSV with the respective goals of these treatments.

Treatment for RSV	Goal
A. mechanical ventilation _____	1. treat RSV
B. bronchodilators _____	2. maintain fluid intake until feeding resumes
C. intravenous fluids _____	3. support ventilatory failure or apnea
D. ribavirin _____	4. relieve airway swelling and obstruction

28. Ribavirin is administered to the patient in aerosol form that is nebulized by a(n)
A. small volume nebulizer
B. large volume nebulizer
C. SPAG unit
D. croup tent
E. IPPB nebulizer

29. SPAG is the acronym for _____
because the particle size ranges from 1.1 to 5 _____ (mm, cm, μm).

30. A full preparation of ribavirin is about _____ (5, 30, 100, 300) mL and it takes about _____
_____ (1 to 2, 4 to 8, 12 to 18) hours for the SPAG unit to nebulize the entire content.

31. If 6 g (6000 mg) of ribavirin is mixed with 300 mL of sterile water, the drug concentration is _____
(0.2, 2, 20, 200) mg/mL.

[NOTES: 6 g (6000 mg) of lyophilized ribavirin is reconstituted with 300 mL of sterile water. The resulting drug concentration is therefore 20 mg/mL (6000 mg/300 mL).]

32. Ribavirin is usually given to a patient with positive RSV culture for a period of _____ (1 to 2, 3 to 7) days.

33. Because of the sticky nature of ribavirin, _____ positive end-respiratory pressure (PEEP) may be a complication when the exhalation valve of the ventilator circuit does not open properly during the exhalation phase of the respiratory cycle.

34. To maintain the proper function of the ventilator circuit during ribavirin administration, the circuit should be changed every _____ hours. In addition, frequent suctioning of the endotracheal tube and use of filters and one-way valves on the circuit may also be helpful.

Concern to Health-Care Workers

35. Because of the teratogen property of ribavirin, health-care workers who are _____ should not be exposed to the ribavirin aerosol.

36. When the ribavirin aerosol therapy is in progress, a tight-fitting _____ capable of filtering out particles down to _____ (0.5, 1, 5) μm should be worn by the respiratory care practitioner (RCP) and other health-care professionals.

37. Side effects of ribavirin may include rash, mild bronchospasm, skin and eye irritation, and headache. (True or False)_____ .

Prevention of Nosocomial Infection

38. In addition to effective handwashing, spread of RSV may be minimized by using all the following prevention techniques **EXCEPT:** _____ .
    A. isolate or dispose of infected or contaminated materials
    B. wear tight-fitting mask
    C. use gloves and gown
    D. obtain RSV vaccine or booster vaccine

CHAPTER **25**

RESPIRATORY DISTRESS SYNDROME IN THE NEWBORN

INTRODUCTION

1. Respiratory distress syndrome (RDS) in the newborn is primarily due to _____ _____ (infection, electrolyte imbalance, prematurity) and it is characterized by progressive
   A. atelectasis
   B. respiratory failure
   C. weight loss
   D. A and B only
   E. all the above

2. RDS is an adverse condition in the newborn that _____ (is, is not) preventable or treatable.

ETIOLOGY

[**NOTES:** Review the table below that outlines the typical events affecting premature infants.]

Events	*Changes in RDS*
Type II alveolar cells	Reduced
Pulmonary surfactant level	Reduced
Lung compliance	Decreased
Work of breathing	Increased

3. Pulmonary surfactant is produced by the _____ (type I alveolar cells, type II alveolar cells, macrophages).

4. Which of the following are factors that limit the amount of pulmonary surfactant produced in the newborn? _____ .
   A. gestational age
   B. birth weight
   C. Apgar score at birth
   D. A and B only
   E. B and C only

5. Pulmonary surfactant reduces the surface tension of the lungs and helps to prevent lung collapse. In premature newborns, surfactant deficiency can lead to _____ (increased, decreased) surface tension of the lungs, _____ (atelectasis, pleural effusion, hyperinflation), and _____ (increased, decreased) work of breathing.

6. Immature lung parenchyma typically produces a _____ (larger, smaller) alveolar surface area for gas exchange, a _____ (thicker, thinner) alveolar-capillary membrane, a _____ (strengthened, weakened) lung defense system, and immature chest wall.

7. When patent ductus arteriosus is present in RDS, _____ (left-to-right, right-to-left) shunt is a common finding because the _____ (left, right) ventricle has a higher pressure than the _____ (left, right) ventricle. This pressure gradient causes shifting of some of its blood into the _____ (left, right) ventricle and eventually the pulmonary circulation. As a result, the pulmonary blood flow is _____ (increased, decreased).

8. If pulmonary congestion is not corrected, interstitial and pulmonary _____ (fibrosis, edema, consolidation) can develop when patent ductus arteriosus (PDA) is present along with RDS.

9. List at least *three* maternal factors that contribute to the development of RDS.

_____

_____

_____

PATHOPHYSIOLOGY

10. Surfactant deficiency causes alveolar _____ (hyperinflation, collapse) and irregular gas distribution. In turn, this condition causes the work of breathing to _____ (increase, decrease) significantly.

11. Progressive atelectasis in RDS is the primary cause of reduced _____ _____ (respiratory rate, heart rate, functional residual capacity).

12. Reduced functional residual capacity causes ventilation-perfusion ($\dot{V}/\dot{Q}$) mismatch in which ventilation is _____ (more, less) than perfusion. This causes a condition known as _____ (dead space ventilation, intrapulmonary shunt).

13. $\dot{V}/\dot{Q}$ mismatch, hypoxemia, reduced surfactant production, and atelectasis are four events that form a vicious cycle of pulmonary deterioration. (True or False) _____ .

MATERNAL HISTORY

14. Sepsis, congenital heart defects, and streptococcal pneumonia are three maternal conditions that can cause respiratory distress in the newborn. The exact cause of respiratory distress should be evaluated and confirmed because treatments for these conditions and RDS are _____ (same, different).

15. Prolonged rupture of the amniotic membrane or fever is a sign that _____ (congenital heart disease, sepsis) is present.

CLINICAL FEATURES

16. Baby Jones, a 30-week-gestational infant, is experiencing respiratory distress 1 hour after birth. When you evaluate this infant, you would expect to see central cyanosis and all the following clinical features **EXCEPT:** _____ .
    A. pulmonary hypertension
    B. nasal flaring
    C. retractions
    D. grunting
    E. tachypnea

17. The breath sounds of baby Jones would be diminished consisting of scattered _____ (stridor, wheezes, crackles).

18. Air bronchogram is a typical radiography finding in RDS. The large airways have a prominent appearance because the _____ (clear, congested) airways are superimposed on the _____ (clear, congested) lung parenchyma.

19. In RDS, the patient's functional residual capacity (FRC) and lung compliance are both _____ (higher, lower) than normal because of _____ (pulmonary effusion, atelectasis, pneumothorax).

20. In RDS, airway resistance is usually _____ (higher, lower) than normal because of the reduction in lung compliance or increase in elastic resistance.

    [NOTES: Resistance to airflow may be imposed by the airways or the lung parenchyma, or both. Airways (e.g., bronchospasm) contribute to the nonelastic resistance to airflow whereas lung parenchyma (e.g., atelectasis) accounts for the elastic resistance to airflow.**]**

21. Baby James, a 28-week-gestational neonate, is diagnosed with RDS. You would expect to see all the following findings in a blood gas report **EXCEPT:** _____ .
    A. hypoxemia
    B. respiratory alkalosis
    C. respiratory acidosis
    D. metabolic acidosis

22. The clinical course of RDS follows a(n) _____ (predictive, unpredictive) sequence.

23. Respiratory distress usually occurs almost _____ (immediately, 2 days) after birth and it peaks in the _____ (second or third, fifth or sixth) day.

24. If surfactant production is adequate, respiratory function usually begins to improve after _____ (1 day, 3 days, 1 week, 2 weeks) and the newborn recovers from RDS about _____ (1 to 3 days, 3 to 5 days, 5 to 7 days).

TREATMENT

25. Because infants of low body weight have a relatively _____ (larger, smaller) body surface area to body weight ratio, they are _____ (more, less) prone to lose body heat.

26. To compensate for excessive body heat loss, infants are able to generate body heat by shivering and _____ (increasing, decreasing) their _____ (white, brown) fat utilization and metabolic rate.

27. To prevent excessive metabolism as a compensatory mechanism for heat loss _____ _____ (thermoregulation, continuous positive airway pressure [CPAP], mechanical ventilation) should be provided to neonates immediately after birth.

28. Thermoregulation can be provided to the neonates by any of the following devices with the **EXCEPTION** of: _____ .
    A. incubator
    B. bubble shield
    C. radiant heater
    D. circulating fan

29. Match the treatments for RDS with the respective goals of the following treatments:

    Treatment

    A. mechanical ventilation _____
    B. indomethacin or surgical intervention _____
    C. oxygen therapy _____
    D. CPAP _____
    E. surfactant replacement _____

    Goal

    1. restore normal surface tension of lungs
    2. provide oxygenation to newborns with intra-pulmonary shunting who are breathing spontaneously
    3. treat hypoxemia in mild RDS conditions
    4. support ventilatory failure or apnea
    5. closure of patent ductus arteriosus

CHAPTER **26**

BRONCHOPULMONARY DYSPLASIA

INTRODUCTION

1. Bronchopulmonary dysplasia (BPD) is a(n) _____ (acute, chronic) lung disease seen mostly in infants who have been on _____ (oxygen therapy, continuous positive airway pressure [CPAP], mechanical ventilation).

2. Conditions that predispose the infants to the development of BPD include all the following **EXCEPT:** _____ .

   A. mechanical ventilation at high inspiratory pressures
   B. mechanical ventilation at high F_{IO_2}
   C. prematurity
   D. A and B only
   E. all of the above

3. The occurrence of BPD is _____ (directly, inversely) related to the infant's gestational age. In other words, prematurity and low birth weight are two factors that are linked to a higher incidence of BPD.

ETIOLOGY

4. BPD is caused by trauma to the _____ (airways, digestive system, lungs) closely related to mechanical ventilation.

5. Use of high inflation pressures and oxygen concentrations in mechanical ventilation may be necessary to ventilate and oxygenate some patients. This may be necessary because of the _____ (high, low) lung compliance associated with conditions such as respiratory distress syndrome (RDS), atelectasis, and shunting.

6. Premature newborns are prone to be affected by _____ (CPAP, oxygen therapy, endotracheal tube) because of their immature antioxidant systems. Because these systems cannot neutralize oxygen radicals during oxygen therapy, lung damage results, particularly at high oxygen concentrations.

7. In infants with patent ductus arteriosus, the pulmonary blood flow is _____ (increased, decreased) due to _____ (right-to-left, left-to-right) shunting of blood. This condition increases the oxygen requirement and risk of oxygen toxicity.

[**NOTES:** In patent ductus arteriosus, the blood shunts from the left ventricle to the right ventricle. This is because the left ventricle has a higher driving pressure than the right ventricle. As a result of this left-to-right shunt, the right ventricle receives its normal venous return from the systemic circulation *as well as* additional blood volume from the left ventricle. This condition causes an increased right ventricular output and pulmonary blood flow.]

8. The increased right ventricular output and pulmonary blood flow may cause pulmonary _____ (embolism, edema, fibrosis). In turn, all the following changes may occur with the **EXCEPTION** of: _____ _____ .
    A. increased oxygen requirement
    B. lower inflating pressures during mechanical ventilation
    C. atelectasis
    D. decreased lung compliance

PATHOPHYSIOLOGY

9. The progression of BPD can be grouped into _____ (2, 3, 4, 5) stages.

10. Match the *four* stages of BPD with the respective key characteristics of each stage.

    Stage of BPD
    A. stage I _____
    B. stage II _____
    C. stage III _____
    D. stage IV _____

    Key Characteristics
    1. pulmonary fibrosis
        hypertrophy of smooth muscle
        destruction of alveoli, airways, and vasculature
        deformation of lymphatic and mucous glands
    2. repair of bronchiolar and alveolar epithelium
        areas of necrosis and emphysema
        airway obstruction and atelectasis
        radiographic signs of opacification
    3. bronchial and bronchiolar metaplasia and hyperplasia
        thickening of basement membranes
        lung emphysema surrounded by atelectatic areas
        increased mucus secretion and interstitial edema
    4. presence of hyaline membrane
        atelectasis
        beginning of brochiolar mucosal necrosis

11. Stage _____ (I, II, III, IV) of BPD is characterized with the presence of hyaline membranes similar to that produced by _____.

12. Match the pathophysiologic changes of BPD with the resultant problems in gas exchange.

    Pathophysiologic Change
    A. atelectasis _____
    B. emphysema _____
    C. increased mucus secretion and interstitial edema _____
    D. air trapping _____

    Problem in Gas Exchange
    1. CO_2 retention
    2. intrapulmonary shunt
    3. dead space ventilation
    4. diffusion defect

13. In BPD, the work of breathing is increased because of progressive reduction of _____ (lung compliance, elastance, airway resistance) and persistent increase of _____ (lung compliance, airway resistance, conductance). In addition, the amount and viscosity of pulmonary secretions are _____ (increased, decreased).

CLINICAL FEATURES

14. During clinical rounds in the neonatal ICU, Dr. Levy asks you to begin trial weaning Baby Jackson off the ventilator. Baby Jackson, a 30-week-gestational infant, has been on the ventilator for about 3 weeks and her current ventilator settings are: FIO_2 = 50 percent, peak inspiratory pressure (PIP) = 35 cm H_2O, respiratory rate (RR) = 36 per minute. Her FIO_2 is changed to 45 percent and the umbilical artery blood gases (ABGs) are as follows:

FIO_2 (%)	pH	$Paco_2$	Pao_2
50	7.36	43	72 (before FIO_2 change)
45	7.38	40	41 (after FIO_2 change)

While Baby Jackson's cardiopulmonary status is stable, the process of weaning should be _____ (continued, stopped) and the _____ (FIO_2, PIP, RR) should be _____ (increased, decreased).

15. Difficult to wean and significant oxygen desaturation with a small drop in FIO_2 are signs of early stage of _____ .

16. As you auscultate Baby Jackson, you hear crackles and wheezes scattered over different lung segments. You may conclude that the crackles signify opening (inspiration) and closing (expiration) of the _____ (atelectatic, consolidated) areas of the lungs.

17. The wheezes heard on auscultating Baby Jackson are indicative of _____ (narrowing, widening) of airways due to bronchospasm or retained secretions.

18. The chest radiograph in BPD may show irregular densities (from atelectasis to fibrosis). In overexpanded areas of the lungs, the radiography resembles that of _____ (asthma, bronchitis, emphysema).

19. Because BPD is a(n) _____ (acute, chronic) problem, blood gas measurements in BPD usually show hypoxemia with compensated to partially compensated _____ _____ .

    A. respiratory acidosis
    B. respiratory alkalosis
    C. metabolic acidosis
    D. metabolic alkalosis

20. In uncomplicated cases of BPD, hypoxemia usually _____ (responds, does not respond) well to oxygen therapy.

TREATMENT

21. Treatment of BPD is primarily _____ (surgical, supportive, pharmacological).

22. Match the supportive measures of BPD with the respective effects.

Treatment	*Effect*
A. bronchodilators _____	1. reduce fluid retention and pulmonary edema
B. diuretics _____	2. support ventilatory failure
C. steroids _____	3. reduce airway resistance
D. mechanical ventilation _____	4. improve pulmonary function

23. Respiratory or ventilatory failure in the newborn is considered present with the following (ABGs) gas parameters:

    pH is less than _____

    P_{CO_2} is higher than _____

    P_{O_2} is less than _____

    F_{IO_2} requirement for the preceding ABG is more than _____

24. One strategy for mechanical ventilation is to use the _____ (highest, lowest) peak inspiratory pressure and F_{IO_2} possible to achieve acceptable ABG values. For newborns with BPD, the acceptable pH should be greater than _____. The P_{CO_2} should range from _____, and the P_{O_2} should be between _____ _____.

25. In the management of ventilator patients who have developed BPD or are prone to develop BPD, weaning from mechanical ventilation should begin _____ (as soon as feasible, on the 3rd day, after 1 week).

26. Use of _____ (CPAP, aminophylline, bronchodilators) in premature newborns with RDS may help to avoid the need for mechanical ventilation and to minimize the occurrence of BPD.

CHAPTER **27**

PERSISTENT PULMONARY HYPERTENSION OF THE NEWBORN

INTRODUCTION

[**NOTES:** In fetal circulation, there are three anatomical shunts (abnormal openings or connections)—ductus arteriosus, foramen ovale, and ductus venosus. Ductus arteriosus and foramen ovale are two shunts that facilitate the return flow of oxygenated blood from the placenta directly to the systemic circulation of the fetus, bypassing the pulmonary system of the fetus. For fetal circulation, see Figure 27-1 in textbook.

Under normal conditions, these three fetal shunts are functionally closed soon after birth. The transitional (fetal to adult) circulation is outlined in the table below.]

Changes During Transitional Circulation

Systemic Alterations (1 to 4)
1. Umbilical cord is clamped after birth
2. Umbilical arteries constrict and close
3. Pressure in left atrium, left ventricle, and systemic circulation increases
4. Foramen ovale closes due to higher pressure in left atrium
Pulmonary Alterations (5 to 8)
5. Lungs begin ventilating
6. Pao_2 increases
7. Pulmonary blood vessels dilate and pulmonary vascular resistance decreases
8. Pressure in right atrium and ventricle decreases
Closure of Shunts (9 to 11)
9. Foramen ovale closes primarily due to a higher left atrial pressure (4 > 8).
10. Ductus arteriosus closes primarily due to increased PaO2 (6)
11. Ductus venosus closes due to vasoconstriction and absence of blood flow

1. Ductus arteriosus is a shunt between the pulmonary artery and the _____ _____ . Foramen ovale is a connection between the right and left _____ _____ .

2. Immediately after birth, initiation of the first few breaths causes the pulmonary blood vessels to _____ (dilate, constrict) as oxygen enters the lungs. This _____ (raises, reduces) the pulmonary vascular resistance (PVR).

3. The reduction of PVR and the concurrent _____ (increase, decrease) of systemic vascular resistance (due to stoppage of placental blood flow after birth) cause the ductus arteriosus and foramen ovale to become closed.

4. In severe and prolonged hypoxic conditions in the newborn, the PVR remains _____ (elevated, depressed) because of widespread hypoxic vasoconstriction in the pulmonary vasculature.

5. If the PVR does not decrease after birth, the fetal shunts will remain _____ (open, closed).

6. When the pulmonary artery pressure (PAP) approaches the systemic artery pressure, the blood flow to the lungs will _____ (increase, diminish) due to a smaller pressure gradient between the left and right ventricles.

7. The condition involving _____ (high, low) PVR, _____ (high, low) pulmonary blood flow, and a fetal state of circulation is called persistent pulmonary hypertension of the newborn (PPHN).

ETIOLOGY

8. PPHN may be caused by any _____ (lung, heart, lung or heart) disease that produces elevated pulmonary pressures.

PATHOPHYSIOLOGY

9. Match the pathophysiologic changes of PPHN with the resultant consequences.

Pathophysiologic Change	*Consequence*
A. decreased pulmonary blood flow	1. shunting of venous blood
B. elevated pulmonary pressures	2. lactic acidosis
C. patency of ductus arteriosus and foramen ovale	3. decreased pulmonary blood flow
D. inadequate tissue oxygenation	4. high ratio $\dot{V}/\dot{Q}$ match

10. The initial stage of PPHN causes the development of hypoxemia and acidosis. These two changes will generally _____ (conclude, further) the progression and advancement of PPHN.

CLINICAL FEATURES

11. Baby Nesmith, a 32-week-gestational newborn, is being evaluated for the presence of PPHN. You would expect to observe all the following clinical signs **EXCEPT:** _____ .
    A. cyanosis with refractory hypoxemia (not responding to O_2 therapy)
    B. loud second heart sound
    C. intercostal retraction
    D. nasal flaring
    E. atelectatic lung segments

12. On chest radiography, baby Nesmith would show lung segments that are _____ _____ (ventilated and clear, secretion filled and congested) but with _____ (increased, reduced) pulmonary blood flow.

13. Preductal and postductal arterial blood gas (ABG) analyses would show a significantly higher Pa_{O_2} in the _____ (preductal, postductal) blood sample.

[NOTES: See question 16 that follows for preductal and postductal ABG analyses.**]**

DIAGNOSIS

14. Differential diagnosis of PPHN may be made by one of three methods. To *confirm* the presence of right-to-left shunt through the ductus arteriosus, _____ (echocardiography, $\dot{V}/\dot{Q}$ lung scan) should be done.

15. The first differential diagnosis of PPHN is done by checking the patient's response to supplemental oxygen. If the PaO_2 is below _____ (100, 500) mm Hg while breathing _____ (40, 60, 80, 100) percent oxygen, it is indicative of significant shunting and suggestive of PPHN.

16. The second differential diagnosis of PPHN is done by comparing the Pao_2 between the preductal and post-ductal blood samples. In the presence of PPHN, a significantly higher Pao_2 would be seen in the _____ (preductal, postductal) blood sample. This is because preductal blood is collected _____ (before, after) the ductus arteriosus shunt and mixing of venous blood.

    [NOTES: In patent ductus arteriosus (failure to close the ductus arteriosus after birth), two blood gas samples are obtained simultaneously—one from the right radial artery (preductal) and the other usually from the umbilical artery (postductal). If transcutaneous Po_2 ($TcPo_2$) monitor is used, a preductal $TcPo_2$ of 15 mm Hg or more than the postductal $TcPo_2$ suggests the presence of PDA.]

17. Preductal $TcPo_2$ may be obtained by placing the monitor pad (probe) on the _____ (left, right) _____ (upper, lower) chest.

18. Postductal $TcPo_2$ may be obtained by placing the monitor pad (probe) on the abdomen or _____ (upper, lower) body.

19. The third differential diagnosis of PPHN is done by performing the hyperoxia-hyperventilation test. The newborn is hyperventilated either by hand or by mechanical ventilation at 70 percent or higher Fio_2. If hypoxemia _____ (improves, fails to improve) with hyperventilation, PPHN is likely to be present.

20. Hyperventilation (respiratory alkalosis) lowers the pulmonary vascular resistance (PVR) caused by PPHN. _____ (Increase, Reduction) of the PVR restores the $\dot{V}/\dot{Q}$ balance and improves oxygenation.

TREATMENT

21. The primary goals in treating PPHN are to _____ (increase, lower) the pulmonary vascular resistance and to _____ (increase, lower) the systemic vascular resistance. This should reduce right-to-left shunting and _____ (increase, decrease) pulmonary blood flow.

22. Match the treatments of PPHN with the respective effects.

Treatments	*Effects*
A. supplemental oxygen	1. treat hypotension
B. hyperventilation	2. dilate pulmonary and systemic vessels
C. paralysis and sedation	3. lower pulmonary vascular resistance
D. tolazoline (priscoline)	4. synchronize mechanical ventilation
E. dopamine	5. treat hypoxemia

23. Extracorporeal membrane oxygenation (ECMO) is the treatment of choice for hypoxemia in PPHN. (True or False) _____ .

24. A nursery resident asks you to explain the respiratory guidelines for the initiation of ECMO. You would explain to her that ECMO might be indicated when the $P(A-a)O_2$ is greater than _____ (100, 300, 600) mm Hg for at least _____ (12, 36, 72) hours.

    [NOTES: $P(A-a)O_2$ equals PAO_2 (calculated) – PaO_2 (measured). The alveolar oxygen tension (PAO_2) is based on an FIO_2 of 100 percent. It can be calculated as follows:

    $PAO_2 = (PB – 47) – (PaCO_2 \times 1.25)$. The arterial oxygen tension (PaO_2) is obtained from an arterial blood sample (preferably from the right radial or umbilical artery in a neonate) when the patient is on an FIO_2 of 100 percent.]

25. If air leak develops during traditional positive-pressure ventilation, _____ _____ (continuous positive airway pressure [CPAP], high frequency ventilation, non-rebreathing mask) may be tried.

CHAPTER 1

ANSWER KEY FOR INTRODUCTION TO PATIENT ASSESSMENT

1. E. A, B, and C.

2. Is not. Assist.

3. The basic methods used during patient assessment should include asking all relevant questions, performing a general examination of the patient to include detailed examination of all sides of the chest wall, and reviewing the chest film.

4. The five basic questions to ask the patient before performing physical assessment are

   When did the problem start?

   Have you ever had this problem before?

   How severe is the problem?

   What seemed to provoke the problem and does anything seem to make it better?

   What region of the body is affected by the problem? If pain is the symptom, exactly where is the pain and does it travel or radiate anywhere?

5. Answers to the questions in 4. will help determine a differential diagnosis, what further tests may be needed, and what initial therapy may be appropriate.

6. The seven common symptoms that may be experienced by patients with cardiopulmonary disease include dyspnea, cough, sputum production, chest pain, hemoptysis, fever, and wheezing.

7. Dyspnea is the sensation of shortness of breath as perceived by the patient.

8. Exertional.

9. Poor.

10. Orthopnea.

11. Heart failure and lung disease.

12. Upright.

13. (1) Mechanical (e.g., foreign bodies, food, liquid, suction catheters). (2) Chemical (e.g., irritating gas, ciga-

rette smoke). (3) Inflammatory (e.g., infection of the larger airways). (4) Thermal (e.g., extremely cold air).

14. Productive. Dry.

15. D. Bronchitis.

16. C. Clear and thick.

17. A. Foul smelling.

18. D. Pus containing.

19. B. Large amount.

20. Sharp. Made worse.

21. Pneumothorax, pulmonary embolism, and pneumonia are three causes of pleuritic chest pain.

22. Centrally. Unaffected.

23. Nonpleuritic chest pain may radiate to the shoulder, arm, jaw, or back; and is more often a dull, pressure type of sensation.

24. Hemoptysis means coughing up blood from the tracheobronchial tree or lungs.

25. Pneumonia, trauma, bronchitis or bronchiectasis, bronchogenic carcinoma, tuberculosis, and pulmonary embolism are some common causes of hemoptysis.

26. Fever.

27. Common respiratory problems associated with fever include viral infections, bacterial bronchitis, bacterial pneumonia, fungal infections, and tuberculosis.

28. Wheezing is a common complaint in patients with asthma, congestive heart failure, and bronchitis.

29. Rapid. Narrowed.

30. Previously.

31. The four basic vital signs are heart rate, respiratory rate, blood pressure, and body temperature.

32. 100. 60.

33. 18. Restrictive. Volumes and capacities.

34. Minute ventilation is a function of tidal volume (V) and respiratory rate (RR). To maintain (or increase) the minute ventilation in the presence of reduced Vt, a higher RR becomes necessary.

35. Pulmonary disorders such as atelectasis, pulmonary edema, pneumonia, pneumothorax, or pulmonary fibrosis cause loss of lung volume.

36. 10. Hypothermia. Central.

37. Decrease. Reduced.

38. Apnea.

39. 120/80. 90/60.

40. Severe hypotension may occur when (1) the heart fails as a pump (heart failure), (2) peripheral vasculature dilates excessively (vasodilation), or (3) the circulating blood volume is severely reduced (volume depletion).

41. 37. 98.6.

42. Increase. Increase. Higher.

43. False.

44. The sensorium level of a patient reflects the adequacy of blood flow and oxygenation of the brain and the net effect of acid or base imbalance, electrolyte imbalance, nutritional deficiency, and other organ system failure.

45. Time. Place. Person.

46. Inadequate. High.

47. Patients with airway obstruction (e.g., asthma, bronchitis, emphysema) tend to breathe with a prolonged expiratory phase, occasionally a prolonged inspiratory phase. Patients with restrictive lung disorders (e.g., atelectasis, lobectomy) use a rapid and shallow breathing pattern.

48. Abdominal paradox is an abnormal breathing pattern seen in patients who have diaphragm fatigue. The abdomen sinks inward with each inspiratory effort when the negative intrathoracic pressure created by the accessory respiratory muscles causes the diaphragm and abdominal contents to be pulled upward into the chest during inspiration.

49. Unilateral.

50. B. Lateral curvature of the spine.

51. D. Anterior-posterior curvature of the spine.

52. E. Increase in the anterior-posterior diameter of the chest.

53. C. Abnormal depression of the sternum.

54. A. Abnormal prominence of the sternum.

55. Consolidated. During verbalization, the vibrations created by the patient's larynx will travel more rapidly through consolidated lung tissue to the chest wall and result in an increase in tactile fremitus.

56. Decreased. Emphysema.

57. With chest palpation, subcutaneous emphysema produces a distinctive crackling sound.

58. Diagnostic chest percussion refers to tapping on the chest wall for the purpose of evaluating underlying lung pathology.

59. Increased. Decreased.

60. Increased.

61. Chest auscultation.

62. Trachea. Loud. High-pitched.

63. Sternum. Anterior. Scapulae.

64. Louder. Turbulent.

65. Normal. Soft. Inspiration.

66. Bronchial.

67. Adventitious.

68. Exhalation.

69. Rhonchi.

70. Inspiration. Partial.

71. Crackles. Rales.

72. Crackles are believed to be produced by two different mechanisms: sudden opening of small airways and movement of excessive airway secretions with breathing.

73. Right. Failure of the right ventricle leads to a backup of blood into the jugular vein (as well as other systemic veins) and causes it to distend.

74. Enlargement of the right ventricle usually results in an abnormal pulsation around the sternum known as a right ventricular heave. Left ventricular enlargement causes an abnormal heave in the left anterior axillary region and is associated with left ventricular failure.

75. Mitral. Tricuspid. Systole. Aortic. Pulmonary. Diastole.

76. S3 gallop. Filling. Diastole.

77. Turbulent. Narrow.

78. Oxygenated. Cyanosis.

79. Hepatomegaly. Right.

80. True.

81. Oral. Severe.

82. Pursed-lip breathing is a breathing technique naturally adopted by patients with chronic obstructive pul-

monary disease (COPD). This breathing pattern creates back pressure during exhalation and helps to maintain patency of the distal airways.

83. 10,000.

84. 5000.

85. White blood cells.

86. Segs. Bands. Segs. Bands. Severe.

87. Anemia.

88. Polycythemia.

89. The electrolyte normal ranges are sodium (Na+) equal to 138 to 142 mEq/L; potassium (K+) equal to 3 to 5 mEq/L; chloride (Cl–) equal to 101 to 105 mEq/L, and total bicarbonate (HCO3–) equal to 23 to 27 mEq/L.

90. Gram stain. Culture and sensitivity.

91. Enzymes. Elevated.

92. Severe.

93. Paco$_2$. Hypoventilation.

94. Below. 7.35. Hypoventilation.

95. Above. 7.45. Hyperventilation.

96. Below. 7.35. Inadequate.

97. Above. 7.45. Excessive.

98. Vital capacity.

99. 80 percent. 60 percent.

100. Air flow obstruction.

101. Chest radiographs are used to (1) determine the proper position of an endotracheal tube after intubation, (2) determine the proper position of a chest tube, (3) determine the proper position of a nasogastric tube, (4) evaluate the lung tissues and related structures, and (5) evaluate the size of the heart.

102. The size of the heart is evaluated by examining the width of the cardiac shadow on the chest radiograph. Normally the heart shadow is less than half the width of the entire chest. Cardiomegaly causes the heart shadow to extend beyond half the width of the chest.

103. Electrical.

104. Atria.

105. Ventricular. Depolarization.

106. Atrial. Repolarization. Ventricular. Depolarization.

107. 0.2. 0.12. Flat.

108. First degree heart block.

109. Internal conduction defect.

110. Ischemia.

111. Cardiac ischemia will cause tall peaked T waves, then ST segment elevation, inverted T waves, and eventually large Q waves when the cells have died.

CHAPTER 2

ANSWER KEY FOR ETHICS IN RESPIRATORY CARE

1. More.

2. C. Life support.

3. Ethics is a systematic study of the moral principles and virtues that may be used to direct a person's decisions and actions.

4. Guidance.

5. True.

6. Family, religious community, culture, education, laws, age, sex, and finance.

7. C. Active euthanasia.

8. A society. Shared by others.

9. Gradually. Frequently.

10. Specific.

11. The AARC code of ethics are as follows: (to be copied from textbook manuscript).

12. False.

13. Self-regulation.

14. A. To guard against conflict of interest.

15. Codes of ethics (1) may omit important norms and virtues, (2) are not extensive enough to anticipate and cover the complexity of all possible cases, (3) cannot conform to the values of a changing society over time, and (4) may present conflicting rules.

16. The codes of ethics may not be able to consider a patient's personal decision. For example, Mrs. W. in the case study shows that her wish to die is not being considered by the codes of ethics.

17. The case of Mrs. W. shows that the codes of ethics cannot prescribe specific solutions for every set of circumstances (e.g., opposing decisions of family members,

use of sedatives to enhance euthanasia, psychiatric exam to determine mental competency).

18. Mrs. W.'s case shows that there is still disagreement about the line between withdrawing life support (i.e., acceptable value of an older society) and ending a patient's life by means of heavy sedation to enhance euthanasia (i.e., newer value of a changing society).

19. Patient confidentiality (e.g., medical history of a child in an intensive care unit) and mandatory report to law enforcement (e.g., suspected case of child abuse) may be two conflicting rules in the typical codes of ethics.

20. Moral dilemma occurs when two or more moral values are in conflict.

21. Two.

22. Broad. Large.

23. Autonomy.

24. D. Personal autonomy.

25. A. Nonmaleficence.

26. Nonmaleficence.

27. Withdraw.

28. C. Beneficence.

29. B. Paternalism.

30. Medical decisions that are made on behavior of young children and mentally incompetent individuals are two examples that show paternalism in health care is sometimes a necessity.

31. B. One desirable effect and one harmful effect.

32. A. Principle of justice.

33. A. Principle of fidelity.

CHAPTER 3

ANSWER KEY FOR INTRODUCTION TO RESPIRATORY FAILURE

1. External.

2. Internal.

3. Carbon dioxide.

4. Respiratory.

5. Oxygenation.

6. $Paco_2$. 45 or 50.

7. Hypoxemia.

8. A. 2. B. 1. C. 3. D. 4. 60.

9. 60. Subtracted.

10. 40.

11. A. 3. B. 2. C. 1. D. 4.

12. At the tissues. In the blood.

13. Increasing.

14. A. $\dot{V}/\dot{Q}$ mismatch.

15. Low $\dot{V}/\dot{Q}$ means the degree of perfusion is greater than the degree of ventilation. It occurs when some regions of the lungs are poorly ventilated but remain perfused by pulmonary blood.

16. High $\dot{V}/\dot{Q}$ means the degree of ventilation is greater than the degree of perfusion. It occurs when perfusion to a portion of the lungs is reduced or absent despite adequate ventilation of the affected region.

17. Intrapulmonary shunt refers to the pulmonary circulation that does not come in contact with the ventilated alveoli. Because shunted blood cannot receive oxygen, it enters and leaves the left heart with highly desaturated hemoglobin leading to hypoxemia in the systemic circulation.

18. Physiologic.

19. Anatomic.

20. Hypoxia or hypoxemia.

21. Decreases. Increases.

22. Fio_2 or oxygen.

23. Decreased.

24. Patent. Compliant.

25. Elastic recoil.

26. A. 2, 7. B. 1, 4. C. 5, 6. D. 3, 8.

27. Low.

28. Hyperinflation.

29. Severity.

30. Increased. Increased. Decreased. Increased.

31. Anatomic dead space is the volume of gases in the conducting airways.

32. Constrict. Vasoconstriction.

33. Increased. Right.

34. Right.

35. Right.

36. Increased. Increased.

37. Sensorium. Coma.

38. Decreased. Increased.

39. Vasodilation.

40. Accessory. Breathing.

41. Cyanosis. Anemia.

42. B. Respiratory arrest.

43. A. Cerebral hypoxia.

44. Increase. Right. D. Bronchospasm.

45. A. 2. B. 2. C. 1. D. 1.

46. Red.

47. Hemoglobin.

48. E. Asthma.

49. C. Hyperventilation.

50. Hypothermia. Loss of consciousnesss.

51. Fixed and dilated.

52. Gag. Crackles. Right.

53. Diaphragm or major respiratory muscles.

54. $Paco_2$. pH.

55. Oxygenation.

56. Oxygen therapy.

57. Moderate. Hypoventilation. Oxygen therapy.

58. Venturi mask.

59. Respiratory rate. Tidal volume.

60. Does not. Shunted blood does not come into contact with ventilated and oxygenated alveoli.

61. Anatomic.

62. Physiologic.

63. Positive-pressure ventilation or PEEP.

64. A. No. B. Positive-pressure or mechanical ventilation.

65. Continuous positive airway pressure.

66. Able.

67. (1) If CPAP does not correct hypoxemia. (2) If CPAP does not decrease the work of breathing. (3) When the medical problem is not likely to resolve soon.

68. Positive end-expiratory pressure.

69. Lower. Oxygen toxicity.

70. Intermittent mandatory ventilation.

71. IMV. Assist control.

72. Inspiratory. Expiratory.

73. Expiratory. Increasing.

74. Lung compliance.

75. Refractory hypoxemia.

76. Pco_2.

77. A. 35. B. 15. C. 10. D. −20. E. 50. F. 60.

78. 10 to 15. 600 to 900.

79. E. B and C only.

80. Atelectasis.

81. 35. 45. Intracranial.

82. A. I and III only.

83. Alkalosis.

84. (1) Prevention of toxin absorption (stomach lavage, emetics, charcoal); (2) enhancement of drug excretion (dialysis); and (3) prevention of accumulation of metabolic end products.

85. A. 10 to 15. B. 10. C. −20. D. 0.50. E. 35. F. 325.

86 Pressure support. Inspiration.

87. IMV.

88. T-piece.

89. Spontaneous.

CHAPTER 4

ANSWER KEY FOR ASTHMA

1. Obstructive. Bronchospasms.

2. Reversible.

3. Status asthmaticus.

4. A. 2, 4. B. 1, 3.

5. Occupational.

6. 1 month.

7. A. 2. B. 1, 3, 8. C. 7. D. 4, 5, 6.

8. B. I, II, and III only.

9. Thick. Plugging or obstruction.

10. B. I, II, and III only.

11. Increases. Decreases.

12. High. Increased.

13. True.

14. False.

15. False.

16. True.

17. Diagnosis.

18. (1) Rapid. (2) Active. (3) Exhalation. (4) Increased. (5) Presence. (6) Retraction.

19. Prolonged.

20. D. II and IV only.

21. Wheezing.

22. Retractions are intermittent depression of the skin around the rib cage occurring with each inspiratory effort. Retractions indicate that the work of breathing is extremely high, caused by airway obstruction or low lung or chest wall compliance.

23. Negative.

24. Inspiration. Paradoxical.

25. Hyperinflation.

26. A. I and III only.

27. Forced expiratory volume in 1 second.

28. 100. 1.

29. Airway reactivity.

30. Increases. Stimulated. Bronchospasm.

31. Decrease.

32. Decreased.

33. Increased.

34. B. I, II, and IV.

35. Bronchodilation. Inflammation.

36. Bronchodilators.

37. Metered-dose inhaler.

38. Convenient.

39. Small volume nebulizer.

40. 4. 6.

41. Theophylline.

42. Hours.

43. Ventilatory.

44. Bronchospasm.

45. Hydration.

46. A. At rest. B. Present. C. Present. D. 100. E. Hyperinflation. F. Accessory. G. Oxygen.

47. A. Increasing. B. Decreasing. C. Presence. D. Decreasing. E. F_{IO_2}. F. Less than 7.25. G. Present. H. Absent. I. Present. J. Unconscious.

48. Decreasing.

49. Avoidance. Medications.

50. Peak flow meter.

51. Mast. Histamine. Bronchospasm.

CHAPTER 5

ANSWER KEY FOR CHRONIC BRONCHITIS

1. Productive.

2. 3. 2.

3. Chronic obstructive pulmonary disease.

4. C. II and III.

5. D. Pneumonia.

6. Cigarette smoking.

7. Infection, air pollution, and occupational exposure to irritants.

8. Larger. Higher.

9. Cilia.

10. Mucus. Cilia.

11. Airflow.

12. Hypoxemia.

13. Vasoconstriction.

14. Constriction.

15. Increase. Hypertension.

16. Increases. Right.

17. Right. Cor pulmonale.

18. Chronic cough. Sputum.

19. C. White or mucoid.

20. Yellow-green.

21. Hemoptysis.

22. A. 3. B. 4. C. 5. D. 2. E. 1.

23. Are. Expiratory. Are.

24. C. Pulmonary edema.

25. C. I and IV.

26. Red. Oxygen.

27. White blood cell.

28. Hypoxemia. Acidosis.

29. Right-sided heart failure or cor pulmonale.

30. Decreased. Increased.

31. Normal. Normal.

32. B. Right axis deviation.

33. D. II and IV.

34. Nicotine.

35. A. Cromolyn sodium.

36. A. Postural drainage.

37. 55.

38. Arterial. P_{O_2}.

CHAPTER 6

ANSWER KEY FOR EMPHYSEMA

1. Obstructive. Dilation. Bronchioles.

2. Including. Deficiency.

3. Excluding.

4. Cigarette smoking. $\alpha_1 PI$ deficiency.

5. Increases.

6. Decreases. Retention.

7. Elastin.

8. Destroys. Increases. Panlobular.

9. Decreased. Decreased. Increased. Decreased.

10. C. Alveolar capillary beds and surface area for gas exchange.

11. D. Low lung compliance.

12. C. Intrapulmonary shunting.

13. B. Prolonged inhalation phase.

14. Forward.

15. Flattened. Small and vertically. Increased.

16. Decrease. Increase. Air trapping.

17. Acidosis.

18. Vertical. QRS.

19. 55.

20. B. Perform complete pulmonary function studies.

21. Important.

22. 55.

23. Bronchodilator.

24. A. 4. B. 1. C. 2. D. 3.

25. Reversible.

26. Prolastin.

CHAPTER 7

ANSWER KEY FOR CYSTIC FIBROSIS

1. Inherited. Bronchiectasis.
2. E. A and C
3. Recessive. 25. 50.
4. B. Renal failure.
5. Diminished. Fibrotic. Obstructed.
6. A. Pulmonary edema.
7. Larger. Increased. Common. Enlarged.
8. D. Epiglottitis.
9. Deficiency of. Diarrhea. Fatty.
10. Salt. Do not. Dehydration.
11. Sinusitis.
12. Malnourished. Accessory muscles. Productive.
13. A. Decreased AP diameter of chest.
14. Cor pulmonale. Right.
15. Increased.

16. Hypoxemia. Hypercapnia.
17. Increased.
18. Increased.
19. Hyperinflation. Flattened. Increased.
20. Decreased.
21. 60. Children. Adults.
22. A. Mycobacterium tuberculosis.
23. Have.
24. D. Antibiotics.
25. Common. A. Change in blood pressure.
26. Gentamicin. Infection.
27. Asthma.
28. True.
29. False.
30. Improving.

CHAPTER 8

ANSWER KEY FOR HEMODYNAMIC MONITORING

1. D. Body tissue.

2. Away from. To.

3. B. Arteries have smooth muscle that can help regulate blood pressure.

4. A. 3. B. 4. C. 5. D. 1. E. 2.

5. Arteries. Veins.

6. Pulmonary. Systemic.

7. Hypertensive crisis.

8. Left.

9. 4 to 8.

10. Body size. Cardiac output and body surface area.

11. 2.5 to 4.

12. Heart rate. HR.

13. Sympathetic. Parasympathetic.

14. A. Cardiac index.

15. Preload.

16. Decreased. Decreased.

17. CVP. PCWP.

18. Within normal limits.

19. Higher than normal.

20. Afterload.

21. Systemic artery. Mean arterial pressure (MAP). Right atrium. Central venous pressure (CVP).

22. Pulmonary artery. Pulmonary artery pressure (PAP). Left atrium. Pulmonary capillary wedge pressure (PCWP).

23. (MAP − CVP) × 80/CO. (PA − PCWP) × 80/CO.

24. Drop. Shock.

25. Contractility.

26. Cardiac output.

27. Preload and afterload.

28. Reduce.

29. Raise.

30. Shock.

31. A. 2. B. 3. C. 1.

32. Obstructed. Inadequate.

33. Septic shock.

34. Microorganisms.

35. A. 3. B. 2. C. 1.

36. Left. Edema.

37. Adult respiratory distress syndrome (ARDS).

38. E. High blood pressure.

39. C. Increased urine output.

40. Acidosis.

41. Lower.

42. NaCl.

43. 8 to 16. 16.

44. Lower. White.

45. Increased. Decreased. Low to normal.

46. Decrease.

47. Poor. Cool. Slow. Is.

48. Tachycardia. Excessive.

49. Coronary.

50. Hypotension. Afterload.

51. A. 3. B. 4. C. 1. D. 2.

52. Hypovolemic.

53. 90.

54. Does. Pulmonary artery.

55. Septic. Microorganisms.

56. Dopamine.

CHAPTER 9

ANSWER KEY FOR PULMONARY THROMBOEMBOLIC DISEASE

1. Blood serum.

2. Blood vessels. Thrombi.

3. Hypercoagulability, damage to the endothelial wall of blood vessels, and venostasis are the three main causes for the formation of venous thrombi.

4. B. Hypercoagulability factors.

5. C. Damage to the venous blood vessels.

6. Slowed venous blood flow.

7. Choose any five of seven risk factors: obesity, congestive heart failure, malignancy, burns, use of estrogen-containing drugs, postoperative state, and postpartum state.

8. C. Deep veins of the lower extremities.

9. Dead space ventilation. Ventilation. Perfusion.

10. Decrease. Atelectasis.

11. A. Increase of lung compliance.

12. A. Vasoconstriction induced by hypoxia.

13. B. Increasing the right ventricular function.

14. Diminishes. Hypotension.

15. 50.

16. Greater.

17. Destruction. Shortly.

18. False.

19. Transient dyspnea.

20. E. Systemic hypertension.

21. Inadequate.

22. Symptoms of pulmonary thromboembolism in the order of occurrence are dyspnea, pleuritic pain, cough, leg swelling, leg pain, hemoptysis, palpitations, wheezing, and angina-like pain.

23. Signs of pulmonary thromboembolism in the order of occurrence are tachypnea, crackles, tachycardia, increased P2, diaphoresis, fever, pleural friction rub, and cyanosis.

24. 20. 100.

25. Right.

26. Venous.

27. Sometimes.

28. Infarction.

29. Normal findings.

30. Closure. Increased PVR.

31. A. High. B. High. C. Normal to low.

32. Pulmonary. Inadequate.

33. High.

34. Alkalosis. Mild to moderate. Increased.

35. Tachycardia. Occasional.

36. C. Rule out pulmonary embolism.

37. Ventilation. Perfusion. Normal. Decreased.

38. Two. One.

39. Angiography.

40. D. Intravenous heparin.

41. Prevent the formation of new clots.

42. Dissolve the existing clots. B. Urokinase and streptokinase.

43. High F_{IO_2}. Mechanical ventilation.

44. D. II and III only.

45. B. Early ambulation and use of elastic stockings.

46. C. Coronary artery disease.

CHAPTER 10

ANSWER KEY FOR HEART FAILURE

1. D. 50.

2. D. Multiple organ failure, perfusion loss, and stasis.

3. Right. Chronic pulmonary disease.

4. A. Hypertension and coronary artery disease.

5. A. 1. B. 2. C. 2. D. 1. E. 1. F. 2. G. 1.

6. Product.

7. $\dot{Q}_T = HR \times SV$.

8. Heart rate.

9. Stroke volume.

10. A balanced output.

11. Thicker. A. Sustaining a higher workload than the right heart.

12. Left. Right. Left.

13. Decreases.

14. 70.

15. Ventricles. Heart beat.

16. Is. 70.

17. C. Stimulation of the β-receptors of the heart pacing system.

18. A. End-diastolic filling volumes.

19. Coronary arteries.

20. Tachycardia.

21. End-diastolic.

22. Greater. Less.

23. Increased. Dilation.

24. Decrease. Reduce.

25. Chronic. A. I and II only.

26. Decrease. Increases.

27. From A to B.

28. Increased.

29. Low.

30. Hypoperfusion.

31. Hyperperfusion.

32. True.

33. Decreased.

34. Reduced. Angiotensin I and II.

35. Reabsorption. High. Retention.

36. Pulmonary and systemic.

37. Outward.

38. Lymphatic.

39. Interstitial. Increase. Increase. Decrease.

40. 25. 5.

41. A. Increase perfusion to poorly perfused areas.

42. A. Decrease in lung volumes.

43. Acidosis. Hypoventilation. Anaerobic.

44. A. 2. B. 3. C. 1.

45. D. Reduced work of breathing.

46. Reduction.

47. Congestion. Jugular.

48. Pitting.

49. Orthopnea.

50. Higher.

51. Reduced.

52. Crackles. Wheezes.

53. Airway narrowing in congestive heart failure is caused by vascular compression of the airways.

54. Large. Excessive.

55. Hypertension. Distension.

56. Widened.

57. 50.

58. Hilum.

59. Pleural surface.

60. C. PCWP of 18 mm Hg.

61. A. Ventricular fibrillation.

62. C. Severe left heart failure.

63. Larger. Reduced.

64. Respiratory. Metabolic.

65. Oxygen.

66. Sodium. Potassium.

67. Bilirubin.

68. Impairment.

69. B. Anatomic changes of the heart.

70. Vasodilators.

71. Salt.

72. D. Relieving pulmonary edema by diuresis.

73. C. 15 to 18.

74. 1 day.

75. C. Improving cardiac contractility.

76. C. Digitalis level.

77. Digitalis.

78. A. Dead space ventilation.

79. C. Reduction of lung compliance.

80. B. Intubation and mechanical ventilation.

81. B. Initiate positive end-expiratory pressure (PEEP) of 5 cm H_2O.

82. B. Aerosolized bronchodilator.

CHAPTER 11

ANSWER KEY FOR SMOKE INHALATION AND BURNS

1. D. Mortality rate.

2. C. Sensory functions.

3. Three.

4. A. 1, 9. B. 2, 3, 6, 8, 11. C. 4, 5, 7, 10.

5. B. Fewer house fires.

6. C. Both A and B.

7. Air.

8. 500.

9. Respiratory irritants.

10. 5. 10.

11. Incomplete. B. Lack of oxygen.

12. A. Plastics containing polyvinyl chloride.

13. D. Polyurethane materials such as nylon.

14. 0.1 to 5. 30.

15. (1) Absorbed, producing systemic toxic effects.
    (2) Deposited, producing local inflammatory changes.

16. D. Heart.

17. Strong. Less.

18. A. Percent.

19. Enhances. Decreasing.

20. True.

21. D. II and IV only.

22. 60.

23. C. Switching the tissues into anaerobic metabolism.

24. C. I and III only.

25. B. I, II, and III only.

26. Blistering, edema, and accumulation of thick saliva.

27. B. II, III, and IV only.

28. C. Loss of a patent airway.

29. D. I, III, IV, and V.

30. C. Increased bronchial blood flow.

31. A. Increase. B. Decrease. C. Increase. D. Increase.

32. A. Increase. B. Increase. C. Increase. D. Decrease.

33. From.

34. A. Overall edema.

35. Decreased.

36. Decrease. Decrease. Ventilatory failure.

37. Decreasing. Increasing.

38. Increased.

39. Increased.

40. Fluid. Increased.

41. Increased. Hindered.

42. Small airways.

43. Atelectasis and airway obstruction.

44. Decrease.

45. C. Bacterial infections.

46. Decrease. Increase.

47. Increased. Tachycardia.

48. High. Weeks.

49. Multiorgan failure. Sepsis.

50. Increased.

51. High.

52. Pneumonia.

53. D. III and IV.

54. Co-oximetry.

55. 60.

56. C. Higher than actual O_2 saturation value.

57. Suggest.

58. Upper airway.

59. More.

60. Rarely.

61. $FEF_{25-75\%}$. Peak flow.

62. Greater than. Less than.

63. Alkalosis. Acidosis.

64. B. Rule of nines.

65. A. Second. B. First. C. Third.

66. (1) Maintain a patent airway. (2) Effective ventilation. (3) Adequate oxygenation. (4) Acid and base balance. (5) Cardiovascular stability. (6) Maintenance of lung volumes. (7) Suppression of infection.

67. D. Work of breathing.

68. Bronchodilator.

69. C. Not preferred because of infections and high mortality rates.

70. (1) Minimize early pulmonary edema. (2) Maintain lung volume. (3) Support edematous airways. (4) Optimize $\dot{V}/\dot{Q}$ matching.

71. C. Receive 100 percent oxygen via non-rebreathing mask until Hbco levels are less than 10 percent.

72. B. Mask CPAP with 100 percent F_{IO_2}.

73. E. Respiratory alkalosis.

74. C. Increasing the removal rate for Hbco.

75. Acidosis. Hypoxemia. 60.

76. Airway plugging.

77. 30 to 50. 2 to 6.

78. Prevents.

79. Compliance. Compressive.

80. (1) Application of topical antibiotic dressings. (2) Wound closure with temporary skin substitutes. (3) Grafting of skin from unburned areas and cloned skin.

81. C. Prophylactic corticosteriods.

CHAPTER 12

ANSWER KEY FOR NEAR DROWNING

1. 85 to 90. 10 to 15.

2. B. And survives for at least 24 hours.

3. Alcohol.

4. Hypoxia.

5. Ischemia.

6. 2. 4 to 6.

7. Bradycardia. Vasoconstriction.

8. (1) Digestion—fat (fatty acid)—fat breakdown (β-oxidation). (2) Digestion—carbohydrate (glucose)—glycolysis. (3) Digestion—protein (amino acids)—gluconeogenesis.

9. D. Glycolysis produces a net of 2 ATP compared with 36 under aerobic conditions.

10. B. Cellular distension.

11. D. Volume, type, and components of the aspirate.

12. Freshwater. Enters. Collapse.

13. Salt water. Draws fluid from. Collapse.

14. D. I, III, IV, and V.

15. Inflammatory. A. Pleural effusion.

16. B. Noncardiogenic pulmonary edema.

17. A. 2, 5, 8. B. 1, 4, 6. C. 3, 7.

18. Hypoxia.

19. Acute tubular necrosis.

20. (1) Length of submersion. (2) Type of fluid involved. (3) Vital signs on removal from the water. (4) Length of time between submersion and CPR. (5) How long was CPR performed before return of vital signs. (6) Water temperature. (7) Age of victim. (8) Alcohol, drug involvement.

21. C. Patient's Po_2 level.

22. Bradycardia. Asystole.

23. Dilated. Slow to nonreactive.

24. A. 3. B. 1. C. 2.

25. D. Skin that is cool to the touch.

26. B. Metabolic acidosis.

27. Freshwater.

28. A. Silverman-Anderson scale.

29. A total Glasgow coma score of 7 or less indicates the presence of coma.

30. 2. 2. 3. 7. Presence.

31. (1) Age 3 years or under. (2) Estimated submersion time longer than 5 minutes. (3) No resuscitative measures attempted for at least 10 minutes. (4) Patient comatose on arrival at the hospital. (5) Arterial blood pH 7.10 or lower.

32. 3. Poor.

33. C. Category C.

34. Out of the water.

35. Should not.

36. B. I and IV.

37. Neck fracture.

38. 60. Chest radiograph. Bronchodilators. Intravenous.

39. A. Hypocapnia.

40. E. Dilated pupils and nonreactive to light.

41. Should. Antibiotics.

42. E. Vitamin K.

43. When culture results are positive.

44. 320. mOsm/L.

45. 7.

46. (1) Normal ventilation. (2) Oxygenation. (3) Perfusion. (4) Blood pressure. (5) Blood sugar. (6) Electrolyte levels.

47. Pulmonary edema. Intracranial pressure.

48. Dehydration by fluid restriction.

49. Increases. Vasoconstricting. Decrease.

50. 25 to 30.

51. (1) Increase tidal volume. (2) Increase respiratory rate.

52. Intrapulmonary shunting. 5. Smaller.

53. B. Hypermetabolic rate.

54. B. Oxygen consumption.

55. D. Seizures.

56. C. May suppress the immune response and cause a higher incidence of infection.

57. Raised. A. Barbiturate use.

58. D. Pressure controlled ventilation.

CHAPTER 13

ANSWER KEY FOR ADULT RESPIRATORY DISTRESS SYNDROME

1. Failure. Alveolar-capillary membrane. Increases. Edema.

2. Noncardiogenic. Is not.

3. D. Humoral system.

4. B. Hyperventilation.

5. Alveolar. 24 hours.

6. C. II, I, and III.

7. 7 days. A. thickening of alveolar septa.

8. Edema. Hemorrhagic.

9. Vasoconstriction. Increased. Reversible.

10. Regeneration.

11. 3 to 4 weeks. Collagenous tissues. Thickening.

12. Increased. Hypertension.

13. Decreases. Decrease. Decreased. Increased.

14. Intrapulmonary shunting. Ventilation. Perfusion.

15. Does not. Refractory.

16. Increase. Hypertension. Right.

17. Increase. Tachycardia. Tachypnea. Normal.

18. Increased. Hyperventilates. Alkalosis.

19. Edema. Crackles. Severe.

20. Respiratory and metabolic. Hypoventilation. Anaerobic.

21. A. Minimal abnormalities.

22. E. All the above.

23. Clear.

24. Pulmonary. Artery.

25. Normal to low. High.

26. B. Pulmonary lavage.

27. Infection. Hypotension.

28. Cannot. Intrapulmonary shunting. PEEP.

29. E. Neurological function.

30. Shunting. Decreasing.

31. Decreased. Decreased. Increased. Increased.

32. Pulmonary artery pressure. Artery.

33. 0.6. Decrease.

34. PEEP.

35. 0.4. 5.

36. Changes in blood pressure. Increase in heart rate and respiratory rate. Fall in pulse oximeter O_2 saturation. Decreased mental function.

37. Pulmonary artery.

38. A. 3. B. 4. C. 1. D. 2.

39. Lungs and chest wall. Airways and lungs and chest wall.

40. Decrease. Decrease.

41. Have little or no change. Decrease.

CHAPTER 14

ANSWER KEY FOR CHEST TRAUMA

1. Trauma-related deaths.

2. A. 3. B. 2. C. 1. D. 4.

3. A. 1, 3. B. 2, 4, 5.

4. Subcutaneous. Under the skin.

5. B. Tension pneumothorax.

6. E. All the above

7. Higher. Older.

8. Ribs 1 and 2.

9. Posterior. Midaxillary.

10. A. Pleural effusion.

11. 9 through 11.

12. (1) Hemopneumothorax. (2) Flail chest. (3) Pulmonary contusion. (4) Cardiac contusion. (5) Abdominal injuries.

13. C. Abdominal injuries.

14. Flail chest. Contracts. Expands. Paradoxical.

15. Decreasing. Increasing.

16. A. 2. B. 3. C. 1.

17. Broken ribs.

18. Reduce.

19. D. Increased $\dot{V}/\dot{Q}$ mismatch.

20. 30.

21. Air leak.

22. Blunt.

23. Penetrating chest trauma.

24. B. II and III only.

25. C. Vocal cord damage.

26. (1) Subcutaneous emphysema. (2) Hoarseness. (3) Tracheal deviation. (4) Difficulty in swallowing. (5) Laryngeal tenderness.

27. 70 to 80. B. Computerized tomography (CT) scan.

28. Penetrating.

29. Cardiac tamponade.

30. Myocardial contusion. Elevation.

31. C. Aortic rupture.

32. Penetrating. Bowel. Surgical closure.

33. C. II and V.

34. B. Blood pressure. C. Symmetrical chest movement. D. Breath sounds. E. Breath efforts. H. Presence of subcutaneous emphysema.

35. 12. 3.

36. 12. 4. 10.

37. B.

38. C. I and III.

39. (1) Allows positive-pressure ventilation. (2) Facilitates endotracheal suctioning. (3) Protects the lungs from aspiration.

40. C. Cricothyrotomy.

41. B. Pao_2 less than 80 mm Hg.

42. D. SIMV. 15. 800. 1. 1:3.

43. Hypotension.

44. Increased. D. Pressure-controlled IRV.

45. B. Pediatric patients.

46. A. 3. B. 2. C. 1.

CHAPTER 15

ANSWER KEY FOR POSTOPERATIVE ATELECTASIS

1. D. Collapsed regions of the lung.

2. A. History of chronic obstructive pulmonary disease (COPD).

3. Negative. Larger.

4. Lack of strength.

5. Thoracic cage.

6. C. Hemidiaphragms.

7. Deep breathe and cough.

8. Negative. Vital capacity.

9. A. Restricts chest wall movement.

10. Relaxed. Upward. Limits.

11. B. Upper abdominal surgery.

12. B. Inadequate diaphragmatic movement.

13. C. Overhydration during anesthesia.

14. Rapidly.

15. C. Positive pressure ventilation.

16. E. A and C only.

17. Ventilation.

18. Higher. Overinflation.

19. Lung compliance.

20. Lung infection.

21. A. 3. B. 1. C. 2.

22. Increase. Decreased.

23. C. Atelectasis on the left side.

24. Hypoxemia. Alkalosis.

25. Spirometry. Poor.

26. Assessing the effectiveness.

27. D. A and B only.

28. Refractory hypoxemia. Oxygen therapy.

29. 10 to 15.

30. Chest physiotherapy.

31. Retained secretions.

32. D. Cyanosis.

CHAPTER 16

ANSWER KEY FOR INTERSTITIAL LUNG DISEASE

1. Inflammation. Lower.

2. B. Tuberculosis.

3. A. Histoplasmosis.

4. (1) Cancer chemotherapy. (2) Oxygen therapy. (3) Radiation therapy.

5. B. Inflammation. D. Pulmonary fibrosis.

6. Inorganic.

7. Antigens.

8. C. *Thermophilic actinomycetes.*

9. (A) Air conditioner and humidifier. (B) Mushroom compost. (C) Grain.

10. False.

11. Cancer chemotherapy.

12. A. 3. B. 4. C. 1. D. 2. E. 6. F. 5.

13. Inflammation. A. An influx of immune cells into the alveoli and alveolar walls.

14. Type I. Type II.

15. B. Do not participate in gas exchange.

16. A. Restrictive lung disease.

17. Initial.

18. D. Pulmonary hypertension and right heart failure.

19. C. II, III, and IV.

20. False.

21. Increases. Hypercapnia.

22. Restrictive. Decreasing.

23. Unchanged.

24. Decreased.

25. Reduction. Early.

26. Rare. D. Incease in $\dot{V}/\dot{Q}$ mismatch.

27. C. II and IV.

28. Inflammation. Evaluate the effectiveness of therapy.

29. B. Fiberoptic bronchoscopy.

30. Immunosuppressives. Inflammation.

31. Often.

CHAPTER 17

ANSWER KEY FOR NEUROMUSCULAR DISEASES

1. E. Cardiovascular system.

2. Central nervous.

3. Respiratory muscles.

4. Chemoreceptors.

5. Any one.

6. Medulla. Pons.

7. Rhythmic respiratory pattern.

8. D. A and B only.

9. A. 2. B. 3. C. 1 and 4.

10. C. Chemoreceptors.

11. Oxygen.

12. Central.

13. B. Carbonic acid.

14. Bicarbonate. Hydrogen. Carbon dioxide. Central chemoreceptors. Carbon dioxide.

15. A. 1. B. 3. C. 2.

16. Synapse is the location at which the nerve impulse and the muscle meet (neuromuscular junction).

17. Acetylcholine.

18. Contract.

19. (1) Diaphragm. (2) External intercostals. (3) Scalene. (4) Sternocleidomastoid.

20. (1) Internal intercostals. (2) Abdominal internal oblique. (3) Abdominal external oblique. (4) Transverse abdominous.

21. B. Central sleep apnea.

22. C. Primary alveolar hypoventilation. Can.

23. A. Sedative and narcotic drugs.

24. Below.

25. A. 5. B. 3. C. 4. D. 1. E. 2.

26. Phrenic.

27. Poliomyelitis.

28. ALS. Lou Gehrig's.

29. Guillain-Barré syndrome.

30. A. Failure of the nerve to release acetylcholine. B. Destruction of the acetylcholine. C. Blockage of breakdown of acetylcholine.

31. A. Congenital abnormality.

32. A. Lung volume decrease. B. Respiratory rate increases. C. dyspnea on exertion.

33. (1) Poor cough. (2) Inability to clear secretions.

34. Expiratory muscles.

35. Decreased. Increased.

36. A. 1.5 L.

37. B. Less than –20 to –30 cm H_2O.

38. To perform the MIP maneuver, the patient should exhale to residual volume and then inhale maximally against a closed mouthpiece.

39. Good.

40. D. Guillain-Barré syndrome.

41. A. Myasthenia gravis.

42. B. ALS.

43. C3.

44. Above C3. 20.

45. Between C3 and C8. Improve.

46. Below C8. Atelectasis.

47. D. Long-term mechanical ventilation.

48. (1) Postural drainage. (2) Cough assistance. (3) Aerosol therapy.

49. A. 15. B. 30. C. Increasing.

50. B. Tracheostomy.

51. Heparin.

52. A. 1.5.   B. –30.   C. 300.

53. Unlikely.

54. Supportive measures.

55. B. Threat of respiratory failure is life threatening.

56. Difficulty in swallowing and breathing. Neostigmine. Anticholinesterase.

57. C. Negative-pressure ventilator (body respirator).

58. A negative-pressure ventilator (body respiratory) does not require an artificial airway, thus reducing the incidence of infection.

59. C3. C3.

CHAPTER 18

ANSWER KEY FOR BACTERIAL PNEUMONIA

1. Lung parenchyma. E. All the above.

2. Bacterial.

3. B. Nosocomial deaths.

4. (1) Chronic lung disease. (2) Cigarette smoking. (3) Drug abuse.

5. E. All the above

6. A. Pneumonia.

7. *Pneumocystis carinii.*

8. B. Exocrine system.

9. A. Sleep apnea.

10. B. I and IV.

11. Necrotizing.

12. C. Decrease of shunting.

13. C. Increase in lung volumes.

14. B. Bradycardia.

15. Tachycardia. Tachypnea. Low. Increased.

16. Common. B. Decreased compliance.

17. A. 1 and 4. B. 3. C. 2.

18. Pleural friction rub.

19. Leukocytosis. Worsening. Leukopenia.

20. A. 2. B. 1. C. 3.

21. Respiratory. Alkalosis. Hypoxemia.

22. Before. The antibiotic may mask the type and severity of infection in a sputum sample.

23. Gram's stain allows rapid selection of broad-spectrum antibiotics based on the general characteristics of the pathogens (Gram-positive or Gram-negative).

24. Culture and sensitivity.

25. (1) Fluid therapy. (2) Nutritional support. (3) Oxygen therapy for hypoxemia. (4) Aerosol or humidity to mobilize secretions.

26. A. 1. B. 2. C. 1.

27. Negative. Hand.

28. Sterile.

CHAPTER 19

ANSWER KEY FOR PNEUMONIA IN THE IMMUNOCOMPROMISED PATIENT

1. Easy.

2. Opportunistic infections are caused by organisms that do not usually affect people with a healthy immune system.

3. (1) Ability to differentiate self from nonself. (2) Specificity. (3) Memory.

4. Host. Autoimmune.

5. Antigens.

6. Immune.

7. Scattered throughout.

8. (1) Lymphocytes. (2) Monocytes. (3) Granulocytes.

9. True.

10. (1) Spleen. (2) Thymus. (3) Lymph nodes.

11. B lymphocytes. Immunoglobulins.

12. (1) IgA. (2) IgD. (3) IgE. (4) IgG. (5) IgM.

13. IgM.

14. IgG.

15. IgE.

16. IgA.

17. (1) Natural killer cells. (2) Helper T lymphocytes. (3) Suppressor T cells.

18. Suppressor T cells.

19. Natural killer cells.

20. Helper T lymphocytes.

21. Cell-mediated immunity.

22. Monocytes.

23. Short lived. Tissue. Long-lived.

24. Polymorphonuclear.

25. (1) Neutrophils. (2) Basophils. (3) Eosinophils.

26. Bone marrow.

27. Neutrophils.

28. Neutrophils are responsible for detecting invading microbes; and phagocytosing, killing, and degrading them.

29. Neutrophils. 500.

30. Eosinophils. Bronchoconstriction.

31. Basophils.

32. More.

33. Increases.

34. More. More.

35. Are not.

36. (1) *Streptococcus pneumoniae*. (2) *Haemophilus influenzae*.

37. X-linked agammaglobulinemia. Selective IgA deficiency.

38. Acquired immunodeficiency syndrome (AIDS).

39. Neutrophils. Less than.

40. Neutropenia is an abnormally low number of circulating neutrophils, usually less than 500/dL.

41. Cancer chemotherapy.

42. Similar to.

43. Cough, dyspnea, and fever.

44. In addition to cough, dyspnea, and fever, patients with pyogenic pneumonia may also experience pleuritic chest pain, production of purulent sputum, occasional hemoptysis, malaise, and recent weight loss.

45. Low. Neutropenia. Increase. Increase.

46. (1) Bacteria. (2) Fungi. (3) Parasites. (4) Viruses.

47. Least. Most.

48. General category: Gram-positive or Gram-negative. *Mycobacterium tuberculosis.*

49. Cell-mediated immunity.

50. Sputum specimens should be collected in the early morning after brushing the teeth and oral cavity, gargling with water, and using a 3 percent nebulized saline solution to induce the specimen.

51. (1) Bronchoscopy with broncheoalveolar lavage. (2) Transbronchial biopsy. (3) Open lung biopsy.

52. Human immunodeficiency virus (HIV).

53. CD4+.

54. 800. 1200. 600.

55. (1) *Pneumocystis carinii.* (2) *Mycobacterium avium* complex. (3) *Candida albicans.*

56. (1) Bacterial infections. (2) Tuberculosis. (3) Coccidioidomycosis. (4) Histoplasmosis.

57. (1) Kaposi's sarcoma. (2) Lymphoma.

58. (1) Fever. (2) Chills. (3) Malaise. (4) Weight loss. (5) Lymphadenopathy. (6) Dyspnea on exertion. (7) Productive cough. (8) Pleuritic chest pain.

59. White. Fungus. *Candida albicans.*

60. Because the donor organ is not genetically identical to the recipient failing organ, transplant rejection occurs when a transplanted organ causes the recipient's immune system to attack the transplanted organ.

61. Suppressing. Increases.

62. (1) Nonproductive cough. (2) Dyspnea. (3) Fever.

63. Low.

64. Sensitive. Often.

65. 500. 7.

66. During the period of neutropenia a patient is prone to develop infections because of the small numbers of circulating phagocytic cells are available to fight infection.

67. Infection.

68. False.

69. Empirical treatment is any therapy (e.g., drug therapy) given to the patient based on practical experience.

70. Antibiotics.

71. Trimethoprim. Sulfamethoxazole.

72. Infections due to *P. carinii* are usually treated with a combination of sulfa antibiotics. Intravenous or aerosolized pentamidine may be given to patients who cannot tolerate sulfa antibiotics. Dapsone, primaquine, atovaquone, and trimetrexate have also been used to treat infections caused by *P. carinii.*

73. Amphotericin B. Imidazoles.

74. Mild.

75. (1) Isoniazid. (2) Rifampin. (3) Pyrazinamide. (4) Ethambutol.

76. (1) Isoniazid. (2) Rifampin.

77. Prophylactic antibiotic therapy is used to prevent pneumonia in patients with immunodeficiencies such as AIDS. These patients are at risk of developing several forms of opportunistic pneumonia.

78. Less. 200.

79. Trimethoprim. Sulfamethoxazole. Pentamidine. Dapsone.

80. 100.

CHAPTER 20

ANSWER KEY FOR TUBERCULOSIS

1. False.

2. C. TB infects one new person every minute.

3. C. Ineffective antimicrobial drugs.

4. *Mycobacterium tuberculosis.*

5. *M. tuberculosis* is a nonmotile, nonsporulating, rod-shaped, acid-fast bacillus, approximately 0.2 × 5.0 μm in size. It is a slow growing aerobe that multiplies better in the presence of an abundant supply of oxygen.

6. Aerobe. Highest. Upper.

7. A. Aerosolized droplets.

8. Fomites are objects or material on which the bacteria are present such as clothing, eating utensils, writing objects, and paper.

9. Lymphatic. Circulatory.

10. 6 to 8. Granulomas.

11. Caseation.

12. Ghon. Ghon complex.

13. Difficult. Small.

14. Heals completely. Leaving small.

15. Effective. Not.

16. True.

17. B. TB infection without disease.

18. No. Positive.

19. Live.

20. (1) Aging. (2) Malnutrition. (3) Alcoholism. (4) Diabetes. (5) Immunocompromising diseases. (6) Silicosis. (7) Postpartum period. (8) Gastrectomy. (9) Chronic hemodialysis. (10) Other chronic debilitating disorders.

21. Decrease.

22. Usually.

23. The bronchi may become distorted and dilated when retractions of the lungs occur.

24. Miliary tuberculosis, a disseminated form of tuberculosis, is usually an acute, generalized tuberculosis spread throughout the region or organ system presenting with many small nodules.

25. The ventilation and perfusion *ratio* of a patient with TB is not severely affected because the destruction of infected lung parenchyma (decrease in ventilation) coincides with the destruction of pulmonary blood vessels (decrease in perfusion).

26. Unusual. Unless.

27. Decrease.

28. The medical history of a patient should include recent travel outside the United States, travel of close family or friends who might be infected with TB, nutritional status, immunosuppression, institutionalized care, and previous or current treatment for TB, and exposure of the patient to a person with active TB.

29. (1) Fatigue. (2) Low-grade fever. (3) Night sweats. (4) Chills. (5) Chronic cough. (6) Sputum production. (7) Hemoptysis. (8) Pleuritic chest pain. (9) Weight loss.

30. Are not. Extent.

31. True.

32. Acid-fast smears. *M. tuberculosis.*

33. Use of local anesthetics (e.g., xylocaine) during bronchoscopy can decrease the viability of the *M. tuberculosis* organism. Therefore, use of xylocaine should be noted in the laboratory report.

34. Intracutaneous.

35. Positive.

36. False.

37. Induration of 5 mm or more is considered a positive PPD skin test for persons who have (1) had close recent contact with a patient with infectious TB; (2) had chest radiographs with fibrotic lesions likely to represent old healed TB; and (3) had known or suspected HIV infection.

38. Induration of 10 mm or more is considered a positive PPD skin test for persons who do not meet the pre-

ceding (5 mm) criteria but have other risk factors such as (1) those with other medical risk factors known to substantially increase the risk of TB once infection has occurred; (2) foreign-born persons from high-prevalence countries; (3) medically underserved, low income populations, including high-risk minorities; (4) IV drug users; (5) residents of long-term care facilities; (6) populations that have been identified locally as having increased prevalence of TB.

39. Induration of 15 mm or more is considered a positive PPD skin test for all other persons who do not meet the above (5 and 10 mm) criteria.

40. PPD skin testing is recommended for the following individuals (1) persons with signs or symptoms, or both, suggestive of tuberculosis; (2) close contacts of persons known to have pulmonary TB; (3) persons with medical conditions that increase the risk of TB; (4) alcoholics; and (5) health-care workers.

41. Does not.

42. The 6-month regimen includes a 2-month period of daily isoniazid, rifampin, and pyrazinamide followed by isonianzid and rifampin given daily or twice weekly for 4 months.

43. The 9-month regimen includes 1 to 2 months of daily isoniazid and rifampin followed daily by twice weekly isoniazid and rifampin for the duration of 9 months.

44. Less than 6 months.

45. Hepatitis. Liver.

46. Rifampin.

47. Watching. Take.

48. 9. Under. Over.

CHAPTER 21

ANSWER KEY FOR LUNG CANCER

1. Little change.

2. Primary malignancy originates in the lungs. Metastatic malignancy originates from other tissues.

3. Has. E. All of the above.

4. Twofold.

5. B. Potentiate the carcinogenic effects of smoking.

6. Small cell. Nonsmall cell. A. Bronchocarcinomas.

7. C. Squamous cell carcinomas.

8. D. Adenocarcinomas.

9. A. Large cell carcinomas.

10. B. Small cell carcinomas.

11. C. Hypocapnia.

12. (1) Cough. (2) Weight loss. (3) Dyspnea. (4) Chest pain. (5) Sputum production. (6) Hemoptysis.

13. Initial.

14. D. Electrocardiogram tracings.

15. A. 3. B. 1. C. 2.

16. C. Rupture of the capillaries of the bronchial mucosa.

17. B. Hilar region.

18. Wheezes.

19. B. Partial airway obstruction.

20. A. Tension pneumothorax.

21. C. An organ and is transferred by the lymphatic or circulatory system to another organ.

22. Nonspecific. Poor.

23. A. 5. B. 1. C. 6. D. 2. E. 4. F. 3.

24. (1) Brain. (2) Spinal cord. (3) Liver. (4) Adrenal glands. (5) Bone. (6) Bone marrow.

25. False.

26. 2 to 3 mm.

27. 1 to 2 cm.

28. A. 1.27.

29. Biopsy and histological examination.

30. Cytology means study of the cells. Cytology sample is used to confirm presence of abnormal cell growth.

31. Central squamous cell. Not.

32. (1) Inadequate specimen sample. (2) Degeneration of malignant cell. (3) Purulent samples containing many other cell types. (4) Difficult to distinguish bronchial squamous cell metaplasia from malignancy. (5) Cell lumps produced by asthma patient resemble adenocarcinoma. (6) Difficult to distinguish cellular changes (due to lipoid pneumonia and pulmonary infraction) from malignancy.

33. Not suited.

34. A fiberoptic bronchoscope is an instrument for visual examination of the airways that is capable of going around curves. The scope is connected to a long flexible material composed of glass or plastic that transmits the light along its course by reflecting it from the other side or wall of the fiber.

35. Peripheral and parenchymal. Bronchogenic.

36. Peripheral. Distal.

37. Fluid cytology.

38. B. Select appropriate therapy.

39. Primary *tumor* characteristics. Regional lymph *node* involvement. Distant *metastasis*.

40. A. 3. B. 1. C. 2.

41. A. TNM classification system.

42. Nonsmall cell. A. Stage I.

43. IIIB.

44. Has not. Remission.

45. Primary treatment.

46. Is.

47. Pulmonary reserve. 0.8 L.

48. C. 1.2 .

CHAPTER 22

ANSWER KEY FOR SLEEP APNEA

1. Is not. Insignificant.

2. Mild.

3. 10. 30. 7.

4. (1) Obstructive. (2) Central. (3) Mixed sleep apnea.

5. Obstructive.

6. Central.

7. Obstructive. Central.

8. Hypopnea.

9. Sum. Hypopneas.

10. E. Arterial and mixed venous blood gases.

11. Multichannel.

12. Daytime.

13. Waking. 5.

14. (1) Nonrapid eye movement (NREM). (2) Rapid eye movement (REM).

15. A. 2. B. 4. C. 1. D. 3.

16. A. 3. B. 2. C. 1.

17. Decrease. Decrease.

18. A. Chronic lung disease.

19. Relaxed. Deep.

20. Fall. Rise. Returns. Deeper. Lighter.

21. Deeper.

22. Does not.

23. Vagal.

24. Tachycardia.

25. Systemic and pulmonary. Higher than normal. Higher than normal.

26. False.

27. Daytime. Inadequate.

28. Lateral.

29. A. Productive coughs.

30. A. Skinny built.

31. B. Cor pulmonale.

32. Hypoventilation. Respiratory. Acidosis.

33. E. All of the above.

34. A. 5. B. 3. C. 1. D. 2. E. 4.

35. A. 2. B. 1. C. 3.

36. A. 3. B. 1.

CHAPTER 23

ANSWER KEY FOR CROUP AND EPIGLOTTITIS

1. Narrowing. Increased.

2. Viral. Below. 3.

3. Bacterial. Above. 1 and 5.

4. D. *Haemophilus influenzae.*

5. Below. Bronchi. Laryngotracheobronchitis.

6. Airway obstruction.

7. Increased. Increased. Decreased.

8. Slow. 1 to 2 days.

9. E. A and C only.

10. E. Bradycardia.

11. A. 2. B. 3. C. 1.

12. Ineffective. Viral.

13. Year-round. Bacterial.

14. Cherry red.

15. Swallowing.

16. Airway obstruction.

17. Sudden.

18. Intubation. Airway obstruction.

19. Elevated. Lateral. Neck.

20. Controlled.

21. Before. Antibiotic.

22. Ampicillin. Chloramphenicol.

23. Leak.

24. Good. Improved.

CHAPTER 24

ANSWER KEY FOR RESPIRATORY SYNCYTIAL VIRUS

1. Common.

2. D. A and B only.

3. Fuse together.

4. 4 weeks to 1 year.

5. Maternal.

6. D. A and B only.

7. 2 to 8.

8. Is. Infective.

9. 30 minutes.

10. A. Cell-to-cell. B. Necrosis. C. Edema. D. Airways. Mucus. E. Decrease.

11. A. Plugging or obstruction. B. Hyperinflation. C. Air trapping. D. Decreased. Increased.

12. E. Metabolic acidosis.

13. C. High fever.

14. A. Bradycardia.

15. Work of breathing.

16. Are premature.

17. B. Vesicular.

18. A. 4. B. 1. C. 3. D. 5. E. 2.

19. A. Normal. B. Increase. C. Increase.

20. Decreased.

21. Increased. Hyperventilation. Decreased.

22. Muscles. Hypoventilation.

23. Flattened. Widened. Increased.

24. Interstitial pneumonitis.

25. Respiratory secretions. Nasal washing or swab.

26. As soon as possible.

27. A. 3. B. 4. C. 2. D. 1.

28. C. SPAG unit.

29. Small particle aerosol generator. µm.

30. 300. 12 to 18.

31. 20.

32. 3 to 7.

33. Inadvertent or auto.

34. 8.

35. Pregnant.

36. Mask. 0.5.

37. True.

38. D. Obtain RSV vaccine or booster vaccine.

CHAPTER 25

ANSWER KEY FOR RESPIRATORY DISTRESS SYNDROME IN THE NEWBORN

1. Prematurity.

2. Is.

3. Type II alveolar cells.

4. D. A and B only.

5. Increased. Atelectasis. Increased.

6. Smaller. Thicker. Weakened.

7. Left-to-right. Left. Right. Right. Increased.

8. Edema.

9. (1) Diabetes. (2) Cesarean section. (3) Previous RDS siblings. (4) Second born twin.

10. Collapse. Increase.

11. Functional residual capacity.

12. Less. Intrapulmonary shunt.

13. True.

14. Different.

15. Sepsis.

16. A. Pulmonary hypertension.

17. Crackles.

18. Clear. Congested.

19. Lower. Atelectasis.

20. Higher.

21. B. Respirarory alkalosis.

22. Predictive.

23. Immediately. Second or third.

24. 3 days. 5 to 7 days.

25. Larger. More.

26. Increasing. Brown.

27. Thermoregulation.

28. D. Circulating fan.

29. A. 4. B. 5. C. 3. D. 2. E. 1.

CHAPTER 26

ANSWER KEY FOR BRONCHOPULMONARY DYSPLASIA

1. Chronic. Mechanical ventilation.

2. E. All of the above.

3. Inversely.

4. Lungs.

5. Low.

6. Oxygen therapy.

7. Increased. Left-to-right.

8. Edema. B. Lower inflating pressures during mechanical ventilation.

9. 4.

10. A. 4. B. 2. C. 3. D. 1.

11. I. Respiratory distress syndrome or RDS.

12. A. 2. B. 3. C. 4. D. 1.

13. Lung compliance. Airway resistance. Increased.

14. Stopped. F_{IO_2}. Increased.

15. BPD.

16. Atelectatic.

17. Narrowing.

18. Emphysema.

19. Chronic. A. Respiratory acidosis.

20. Responds.

21. Supportive.

22. A. 3. B. 4. C. 1. D. 2.

23. 7.25. 60 mm Hg. 50 mm Hg. 60%.

24. Lowest. 7.28. 50 to 70 mm Hg. 55 and 65 mm Hg .

25. As soon as feasible.

26. CPAP.

CHAPTER 27

ANSWER KEY FOR PERSISTENT PULMONARY HYPERTENSION OF THE NEWBORN

1. Aorta. Atria.

2. Dilate. Reduces.

3. Increase.

4. Elevated.

5. Open.

6. Diminish.

7. High. Low.

8. Lung or heart.

9. A. 4. B. 3. C. 1. D. 2.

10. Further.

11. E. Atelectatic lung segments.

12. Ventilated and clear. Reduced.

13. Preductal.

14. Echocardiography.

15. 100. 100.

16. Preductal. Before.

17. Right. Upper.

18. Lower.

19. Improves.

20. Reduction.

21. Lower. Increase. Increase.

22. A. 5. B. 3. C. 4. D. 2. E. 1.

23. False.

24. 600. 12.

25. High frequency ventilation.

$$\frac{CcO_2 - CaO_2}{CcO_2 - CvO_2}$$